REINVENTING ACUP

By the same author and publisher

TEXTBOOK OF ACUPUNCTURE.
A traditional textbook with, in addition, 100 pages of research

ATLAS OF ACUPUNCTURE. *Points and Meridians in relation to surface anatomy.*
This is the companion volume to *Textbook of Acupuncture.*

ACUPUNCTURE: CURE OF MANY DISEASES
Second Edition
This is for the non-medical reader who wants a grasp of the essentials of acupuncture in a few hours

REINVENTING ACUPUNCTURE

A New Concept of Ancient Medicine

By

FELIX MANN

MB, BChir (Cambridge), LMCC

Founder of The Medical Acupuncture Society
President: 1959–1980
First President of The British Medical Acupuncture Society (1980)
Deutscher Schmerzpreis 1995

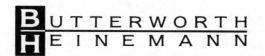

Butterworth-Heinemann
Linacre house, Jordan Hill, Oxford OX2 8DP
225 Wildwood Avenue, Woburn, MA 01801-2041

A division of Reed Educational and Professional Publishing Ltd

ℝ A member of the Reed Elsevier plc group

OXFORD AUCKLAND BOSTON
JOHANNESBURG MELBOURNE NEW DELHI

First published 1992
Reprinted with addition 1996, 1999

Italian edition published by Editore Marrapese, Rome, 1995
German edition to be published Winter 1996. AMI Verlag, Giesson

© Felix Mann 1992

British Library Cataloguing in Publication Data
Mann, Felix
  Reinventing Acupuncture: A New Concept of
  Ancient Medicine
  I Title
  615.8

ISBN 0 7506 0844 7

Library of Congress Cataloguing in Publication Data
Mann, Felix
  Reinventing acupuncture : a new concept of ancient medicine/by
  Felix Mann.
  p.   cm.
  Includes index.
  ISBN 0 7506 0844 7
  1. Acupuncture.   I. Title
  RM184.M353   1993
  615.8'92—dc20   92–27735
                                              CIP

Printed and bound in Great Britain by
Athenæum Press Ltd, Gateshead, Tyne & Wear

Contents

Preface and Acknowledgements

My previous books on acupuncture were largely based on ancient tradition interpreted, to a limited extent, from a Western point of view. They also included research which might be relevant to acupuncture. Thus, these books were essentially the work of others, often unknown ancient Chinese.

This book is the reverse. It concentrates on what I have discovered myself, which frequently contradicts conventional wisdom, both Eastern and Western. All I have done is to *observe and listen to patients* and, at the same time, I have tried to obliterate the preconceptions I have from both Western and Eastern medicine. These observations were thought about, digested, added to 30 years' experience, and then written down as this book. The way I treat patients nowadays and, I hope, help or cure a reasonable proportion, is what you will read in the following pages. I only practise traditional acupuncture, as described in my other books, to a limited extent. Nevertheless, the tradition can be a mine of information for those who can understand it.

Most of all I would like to thank my wife. I had already written books totalling some 800 pages and I had had enough. It was purely her encouragement which started the ball-point rolling again.

The fact that I think differently from many doctors I owe largely to my upbringing. My mother never believed in the conventional: it was boring. She thought about everything in her own way, largely free of preconceptions.

The philosophy and outlook on life of Rudolf Steiner influenced both my mother and myself.

Dr Jean Schoch of Strasbourg taught me to look at patients differently: with the eye of an artist rather than the scalpel of a dissector.

Traditional acupuncture, not mentioned much in this book,

I studied with Dr Anton Strobl of Munich, Professor Johannes Bischko of Vienna and Dr Van Nha of Montpellier. I also learned from many doctors in Peking, Nanking and Shanghai.

Dr Alexander Macdonald, who has done more scientific investigation of acupuncture than anyone else in this country, has been a constant source of inspiration.

David Owen and Frank Liu taught me to read Chinese. This gave me an inkling of the completely different mentality of the ancient Chinese.

I looked through illustrations of medical books for 5 hours until I saw the drawings of the medical artist Mrs Gillian Oliver. These I liked and I hope you, the reader, will do so also.

My wife corrected the manuscript, deleting remarks one can say but not write! Grammar is one of my many weaknesses, which she has corrected as little as possible, as she wishes the style of the book to be mine, not hers.

Mrs Gwen Macnair typed the manuscript, which was a jigsaw puzzle of original text, corrections, corrections of corrections and corrections of corrections of corrections. I was stunned that it needed typing only once.

I would like to thank Mrs Caroline Makepeace for the enthusiasm with which she has taken on something unorthodox. Christopher Jarvis has solved the problem of a difficult text involving different typefaces. The numerous sales staff have coped splendidly with a book which does not fit into a defined pigeon-hole.

Doctors who wish to study acupuncture are welcome to write to me, as I regularly give courses in my practice in Central London. Most of the teaching is done on patients, in a way similar to a teaching ward round at medical school. A different patient is seen every hour; a large variety of diseases is involved. The appropriate treatment is discussed, as well as the chances of success and failure. As these are practical courses they are restricted to about 15 participants, who must be qualified medical doctors.

The courses last 1 week. Greater emphasis is put on empirical results, as described in this book, than on traditional acupuncture.

Felix Mann
London W1

1992

Nomenclature

Traditionally the places which are needled in acupuncture are called acupuncture points: places of small size and fixed position.

In my experience, the places which can be needled are usually *much larger areas, of variable size and position.* Hence in this book I rarely mention the word 'point', preferring instead the word 'area'.

In Chinese the traditional acupuncture points are given names, often beautiful names, such as the 'spirit door' (shen men). Very few Western doctors have learnt Chinese and therefore a numbering system was introduced which, I think, was first used extensively by the French. The 'spirit door', for example, was called 'coeur 7', as it is the seventh traditional acupuncture point on the heart meridian; this was abbreviated as C7.

I wrote what I think were the first comprehensive books on acupuncture in the English language—four books, published 1962–1964. As we had no ready-made English language nomenclature, my Chinese teachers and I largely invented one.

As far as the numbering of acupuncture points is concerned, I largely took over the French system which had in the meantime also spread to Germany, Austria, Switzerland, Italy, Holland and Belgium. Thus I called coeur 7 or C7, heart 7 or H7—a system easily understood in all Western languages. As English is the main international language in medicine, it was inevitable that my numbering system and system of abbreviations became the main international system, that is for non-Chinese readers.

The World Health Organisation (WHO) has recently, at very great expense, introduced another system. This in itself causes needless confusion, in addition to which it disregards basic rules of typography. The ensuing muddle, if it were in the pharmaceutical world, would be disastrous and potentially lethal, but as it is only acupuncture . . . !

In this book I have largely ignored acupuncture points but write instead of *areas*. These areas may or may not include one or several acupuncture points. I have given these areas *anatomical names*, such as sacro-iliac joint area, so that all doctors will immediately know their approximate position. This obviates the need to learn all the acupuncture point numbers and also, incidentally, brings the whole subject more into the twentieth century, given that acupuncture points have no physical existence.

So that all readers may follow the text, most sections are headed as follows:

1 Anatomical name.
2 Nearest acupuncture point name in full.
3 Nearest acupuncture point name in abbreviation.
4 Nearest acupuncture point name in WHO abbreviation.

My step-daughter, a classicist, thought up not only the title of this book, but also the technical words micro-acupuncture and infragenual area. I coined the following terms: periosteal acupuncture, Strong Reactor, upper digestive dysfunction, and the mainly anatomical names, some 25, used to describe the acupuncture areas, such as varicose ulcer area, anterior medial elbow area, etc.

PART I

From tradition to the twentieth century

Acupuncture originated in prehistoric times and evolved into its present form in the succeeding centuries. The vast majority of books on acupuncture, both in the East and in the West, belong to this prescientific era.

Some of these traditional books describe only the skeleton of acupuncture: acupuncture points, meridians and cookbook-like recipes of treatment. The more comprehensive books describe the philosophy and thought processes that underlie this simplified skeleton: yin and yang, the five elements, Qi, Ying Qi, Wei Qi, blood, Jing, Shen, fluid, etc.

The scientific investigation of acupuncture has proved to be extraordinarily elusive, for reasons mentioned later in this chapter. Hence a doctor who wishes to study acupuncture has little to read other than the traditional books.

This book is different. Those who wish to be or to remain traditionalists should read no further, for I will show that many of the major traditional concepts are incorrect, or at least partially incorrect.

According to my concept:

1 Acupuncture points, in the traditional sense, do not exist, though sometimes there are tender areas rather similar to McBurney's point in appendicitis. This is described in Chapter II.

2 Meridians, in the traditional sense, likewise do not exist.

Sometimes, after stimulation, one may have radiation of pain or other sensation which, as often as not, follows a course different from that of the meridians. This is described in Chapter III.

3 I find that the secret of success often depends on administering exactly the correct dosage of acupuncture. This depends on a knowledge of Strong Reactors and Normal Reactors, a concept which is largely alien to traditional acupuncture. This is described in Chapters IV and VII.

4 In my practice I find it necessary to treat the 'liver' in more than half the patients I see, whatever disease or symptom they may have. Perusal of old Chinese books reveals that this was not the case in ancient China. Perhaps this is due to the effect of modern Western civilisation on our health. My contribution to this subject is described in Chapter V.

5 The ancient Chinese or, for that matter, the ancients of most civilisations, did not draw a sharp distinction between the material and the non-material, nor between physical and mental diseases. A marriage of Chinese, Western and my ideas is described in Chapter VI.

6 Periosteal acupuncture, in which the periosteum is stimulated, has a more powerful effect than the traditional subcutaneous or intramuscular acupuncture. I think I invented this, as the ancients allude only fleetingly to periosteal or bone stimulation. It would not have been a practical system as the ancients' needles were as thick as meat skewers or, if thin, easily broken. This is described in the whole of Part II of this book.

7 Also in Part II are described the acupuncture areas, usually large, which have a variable position, rather than the small acupuncture points of fixed position accepted by tradition.

8 My embryonic ideas of a partial explanation of acupuncture in terms of neurophysiology are described in the first hundred pages of my *Textbook of Acupuncture* (Scientific Aspects of Acupuncture).

I had already evolved the above eight groups of ideas within the first few years of starting my acupuncture practice. Since then, I have taught them continuously at the acupuncture courses I hold in London, and also at the mini-courses or lectures I give abroad. More recently I have evolved micro-acupuncture, described in Chapter VII.

In the early years, my ideas, particularly the ones which contradicted traditional acupuncture, were greeted with overt or covert opposition, particularly by the experts in the world of acupuncture. I think most of the ideas were original for, despite giving lectures in 15 countries and teaching doctors from 45 countries at my courses, no experts told me of hearing something similar; nor for that matter could I find much of a similar nature in acupuncture and related literature.

THE DUBIOUS VALUE OF MANY RESEARCH PROJECTS IN ACUPUNCTURE

1 Most research into acupuncture has, as it were, been 'led up the garden path' by the ideas of traditional acupuncture. The researchers have believed in the tradition and then tried to prove it experimentally.

Some have tried to find acupuncture points or meridians by measurement of the electrical skin resistance. Those with a microscope have tried to find specialised structures in the skin or subjacent tissue. Those who have the use of infra-red photography, Kirlian photography or ultrasound have all diligently searched for the elusive acupuncture point. Some have been 'successful' and have described their findings in journals.

If only these researchers had realised that the traditional acupuncture point does not exist!

2 Clinical trials are likewise difficult, for the reader of this book will realise that there is no such thing as a placebo point.

3 The reader of my *Textbook of Acupuncture* will be aware that acupuncture is a strange subject; it may alleviate or cure disease and yet be like a slippery eel when subjected to the standard methods of research.

(a) In cases of, say, migraine, low backache, sciatica or pain in the neck, shoulder and arm, acupuncture will help in a reasonable proportion of patients. A visit to a psychiatrist by patients with these conditions will, on the other hand, result in very few cures. Clearly, acupuncture and psychiatric therapy are not the same, though this does not exclude a partial overlap.

(b) A patient with low backache may have his pain, stiffness and limitation of movement alleviated by acupuncture of the lumbosacral area. Some patients with low backache have electromyographic (EMG) studies of this same lumbosacral area in which EMG needles are often put in much the same area as the acupuncture needles would be. Yet I am told by doctors who do such EMG studies that this investigation rarely helps their patients—admittedly they are usually severe cases.

(c) Migraine may be helped by needling an area on the dorsum of the foot called liver 3. Frequently, however, needling anywhere in the foot may help (though possibly in a smaller proportion of patients). Nevertheless, although a sharp stone in a shoe will stimulate just as much as an acupuncture needle it will rarely cure migraine.

(d) When I started practising acupuncture in this country, it was completely unknown and patients did not know what would happen or what to expect. Several patients thought that the insertion of needles was some sort of neurological test—and not the actual treatment. On several occasions when treating such patients I would ask them, after the insertion of the needles, if their pain, limitation of movement, etc. were any better. I would then receive a reply such as: 'But doctor you have only done the tests, when are you going to treat me?' Upon my insistence that they tell me if their symptoms were alleviated, I might hear: 'Funny—I am cured, but you have not treated me yet . . .'

In this instance the patient was cured in spite of thinking he had not been treated.

(e) If patients are treated too strongly by acupuncture they may experience a temporary aggravation of their symptoms, having, for example, an extremely severe and long-lasting migraine the same evening as the treatment. This is particularly liable to happen in Strong Reactors (see Chapter IV).

Occasionally I do not recognise a Strong Reactor and hence, without my realising it, I overtreat a patient.

The patient obviously does not expect to get worse, nor for that matter do I expect it; yet the patient has what is called a reaction and becomes temporarily worse.

(f) Strong Reactors often have their symptoms alleviated within a few seconds of treatment—which, in the appropriate case, I expect. The patient though, does not expect to be cured in a few seconds, but rather in a few days, being used to orthodox medicine, which usually requires a few days to produce a response.

Despite my expecting one thing and the patient expecting something different, the treatment works—contrary to the patient's expectation.

It is obvious from the examples (a) to (f), and others I could give, that acupuncture is an enigma. It works, but how?

Normally one recognises two states: *health* and *disease*. I think one should recognise three states: *health, physiological dysfunction* and *disease*.

1 *Health* At this stage the patient feels well in every way. All laboratory tests are normal (Fig. I.1).

This is followed by:

2 *Physiological dysfunction* In many cases I think there is a gradual change, which may sometimes take years, from health to disease. The first step along this road is a *mild physiological dysfunction*. The patient is not ill, nor is he well. He may have insomnia, headaches, heartburn, lumbago, etc.

The 'illness' may stay at this level and never become a 'real disease'. The patient may have dysmenorrhoea for 30 years or migraine for 50 years. As the physiological dysfunction is still mild, the laboratory tests remain normal or near normal.

I dare say that, with the refinements of laboratory techniques, one will in the future be able to demonstrate delicate differences at this stage of mild physiological dysfunction. There are, after all, probably a million or more biochemical

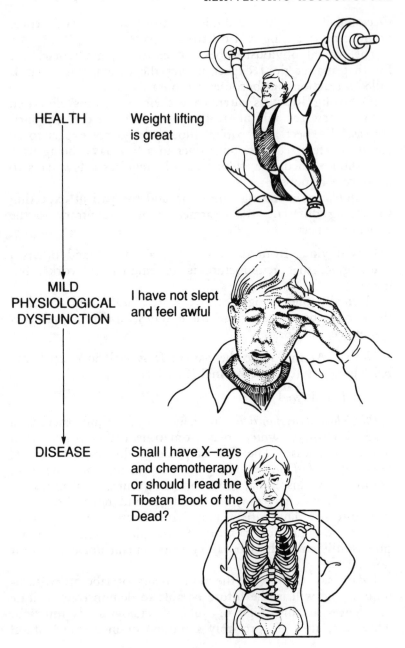

HEALTH — Weight lifting is great

MILD PHYSIOLOGICAL DYSFUNCTION — I have not slept and feel awful

DISEASE — Shall I have X–rays and chemotherapy or should I read the Tibetan Book of the Dead?

Fig. I.1

processes going on in the body. At the moment we can detect some of the more obvious: those that determine life and death. There are probably other less important processes which will be discovered one day and can then be measured.

At this stage of mild physiological dysfunction, where laboratory tests are normal, the doctor can only be guided by a patient's symptoms and his general appearance. For this doctors will have to learn how to *listen to* and *observe* their patients, as doctors did in previous centuries.

This stage is, in some cases, followed by:

3 *Disease* At this stage the patient is obviously ill. The physiological dysfunction has become such that laboratory tests usually demonstrate abnormality. There may even be anatomical changes which can be seen on X-ray. We have now arrived at the stage that orthodox medicine calls 'real disease'.

Generally speaking, acupuncture is of most benefit in those diseases or symptoms which involve a *mild* physiological dysfunction, such as headaches, palpitations or lumbago. In these dysfunctions the pathology is so mild that frequently the patient's symptoms may not only be alleviated, but actually cured, i.e. when the treatment stops, the patient remains more or less cured.

Orthodox medicine is often of greater benefit in those diseases involving a *severe* physiological dysfunction, such as gout, congestive cardiac failure or a slipped disc. As the pathology is severe, often involving an irreversible process, when medication stops the symptoms reappear. Usually only surgery helps permanently or almost permanently in certain cases of irreversible pathology.

The area of application of acupuncture to the diseases involving a mild physiological dysfunction poses some problems. The system of laboratory and other tests used in Western medicine is geared to the Western medical concept of diseases involving a severe physiological dysfunction. The mild diseases treatable by acupuncture often have normal laboratory findings. Patients with migraine or dysmenorrhoea, however, do not look upon their symptoms as mild, even if they are not lethal. Even so, doctors practising acupuncture are often accused of treating diseases which do not exist!

It is also apparent that, in the area of mild physiological dysfunction, the mind and the body may be acting together. The examples above, (a)–(f), demonstrate that sometimes, if there is only the mind or only the body, the acupuncture effect is missing: it requires both the mind and the body to work synergically.

This synergy happens in general practice as well, for the patient goes to a doctor expecting help and the doctor gives a drug which he also hopes will help. In the usual type of clinical trial, in which the patient does not know what is happening and frequently the doctor does not know either, this synergy is missing. This does not matter when administering the powerful drugs used in orthodox medicine, but for something gentle like acupuncture it may make a great difference.

There are many processes in the body that involve the type of mild physiological dysfunction described above, which can be influenced by the mind or the body or, more often, the synergic action of both.

I was once very hungry with, presumably, my digestive juices in full flow. We stopped at a restaurant which was full of dead flies and smelled of manure. My appetite disappeared at once.

On one occasion I had a painful dislocation of the shoulder. When I arrived at hospital the pain was reduced.

In a susceptible person, salbutamol may produce tachycardia and this may produce anxiety. That same person may have a food sensitivity which often also causes tachycardia and then anxiety. Those who have lost a lot of blood due to a haematemesis may notice that the slightest emotion (even watching a Mickey Mouse film on television) may cause tachycardia followed by anxiety.

Acupuncture is, I think, essentially in no man's land, between the land of the mind and the land of the body. A doctor practising acupuncture will have many grateful patients but will be able to demonstrate little objectively. It is a subject full of contradictions, in which the experts often disagree with one another. I derive great pleasure in being able to help, to a greater or lesser extent, a reasonable proportion of the patients I treat—and that is all that the patients ask of me. To what extent I understand what happens is another matter.

For all these reasons and for others which will become apparent in subsequent chapters, it is evident that acupuncture is not a subject that lends itself to bureaucratic control, 'qualifications', etc. As Western scientific and empirical acupuncture emerges from its earliest infancy, the traditional Chinese form will become a field more for medical historians than practitioners. In modern scientific acupuncture, on the other hand, there is as yet no body of agreed scientific knowledge to form the basis of qualifications. Bureaucratisation at this stage would lead to the stifling of originality, innovation and progress.

II

Non-existent acupuncture points

If a Western doctor were to look at certain Oriental or Occidental acupuncture charts, he would see absolutely straight rows of acupuncture points over, for instance, the thorax, abdomen and back. Set at exactly right angles to these are other rows, the whole thing more reminiscent of graph paper than of anything else (Fig. II.1). Traditionally there is even a precise

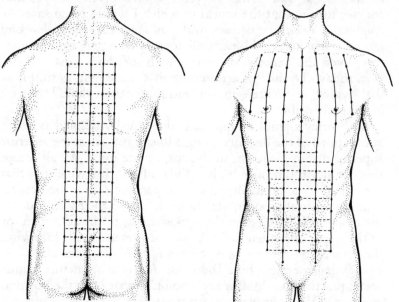

Fig. II.1 The geometrical definition of traditional acupuncture points

system of measurement, which geometrically defines the exact position of each acupuncture point.

We all know that such an exact geometrical system cannot exist in living nature (though it can in inanimate nature, as in crystals), for 'nature abhors straight lines'. There are some acupuncture charts, both Eastern and Western, which are not quite as rigid, though they still depend on a system of measurement or geometry or exact anatomical landmarks. However, later in this chapter I will mention what the ancient Chinese did, which was perhaps nearer the truth than the systems of succeeding generations.

Below I will describe what I think the acupuncture points really are, and I expect to show that, according to one's point of view, they both exist and do not exist; in either case they are something vastly different from what is traditionally described. I think I was one of the first doctors to deny the existence of acupuncture points as traditionally conceived and, what is more, put something else in their place, as described in Part II of this book. For some 30 years I have given lectures and courses throughout the world in which I would often say: *'the acupuncture points are no more real than the black spots a drunkard sees in front of his eyes.'* Nearly all doctors who practise acupuncture, even the experts, disagreed with me, and most still do, even today. To me it is astounding that something as simple as that which is written in the ensuing pages should remain incomprehensible.

McBurney's point in appendicitis is usually defined as being at one-third of the distance along a line drawn from the anterior superior iliac spine to the umbilicus, on the right. We all accept this definition but only with a pinch of salt, for we know that the actual area of tenderness in appendicitis may be several centimetres higher, or lower, to the left or to the right. Indeed, the tenderness may be on the opposite side of the abdomen, or in the upper abdomen or back, or not present at all. Likewise, the area of tenderness may be 1 cm across, 10 cm across or occupy half or the whole abdomen. Many acupuncture points are in practice like McBurney's point, in that both the position and size of the point vary enormously (Fig. II.2).

In a certain type of headache, not necessarily associated with

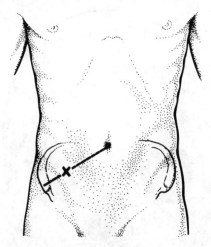

Fig. II.2 McBurney's 'point' is supposed to be at 'X', but it may be almost anywhere. Its size may vary from that of a pea to a dinner plate

a sinus infection, a patient may have a tender area over the medial part of the supraorbital margin, where the supratrochlear nerve arches over the supraorbital margin (Fig. II.3). This area of tenderness is always in the same position and it is also always about 1 cm in diameter. In this respect this place, which is traditionally called bladder 2, is more like the classical description of an acupuncture point. There are, however, few places in the body which nearly always display such a constancy in position and size.

Many patients have a pain in the neck and shoulder associated with cervical spondylosis or osteoarthritis. The tenderness mostly extends from the occiput, along the posterolateral aspect of the neck and across the top of the shoulder, an area, say, 30 cm long and 3 cm wide. Sometimes the whole of this area is affected, whereas at other times only one or several areas within it. Occasionally there may be radiation beyond it (Fig. II.4). It is thus apparent that this cervical tenderness is not as fixed in position and size as the supratrochlear point, yet it is not as infinitely variable as McBurney's point.

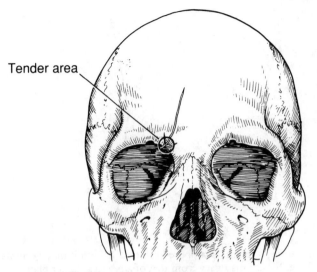

Tender area

Fig. II.3 Tenderness over supratrochlear nerve

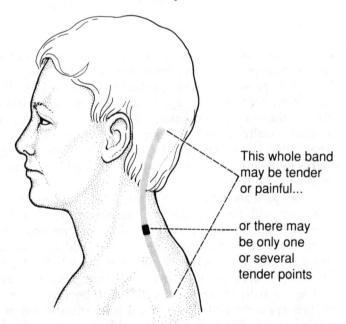

This whole band
may be tender
or painful...

or there may
be only one
or several
tender points

Fig. II.4 Area of occipital, cervical, shoulder tenderness

As far as I am concerned, acupuncture points, if one wishes to call them that, may be just as various as the three points mentioned above. A few are fixed in position and size, whereas others, the majority, are moderately or extremely variable in position and size. Hence, nowadays, I rarely use the word 'point', preferring the more accurate description 'area'.

LOCATION OF ACUPUNCTURE POINTS OR AREAS

The position which should be needled in acupuncture varies considerably in the degree of accuracy required:

1 A needle anywhere—yes, really anywhere—in the body may be sufficient to cure or alleviate symptoms, in certain selected patients. Whenever I mention this at acupuncture conferences the majority of doctors present are either incredulous or antagonistic. I have been asked why I do not stand patients against a wall, close my eyes and throw darts at random. Now, after 25 years of preaching, my views are better known and beginning to be partially accepted (Fig. II. 5).
2 Sometimes a needle anywhere in the appropriate quarter of the body, the relevant arm or leg, is sufficient to alleviate symptoms (Fig. II. 5).
3 Sometimes a needle in the correct or neighbouring dermatome, myotome or sclerotome is sufficient (Fig. II. 5).
4 Sometimes needling anywhere, within an area the size of the palm of the hand, is sufficient. This applies especially often to areas over the sacrospinalis or rectus abdominis (Fig. II. 5).
5 If a trigger point can be found, which is not always the case, and it is needled, the best result may ensue (Fig. II. 5). The trigger point, often about a centimetre in diameter, may, however, only alleviate local symptoms and a general systemic effect may require distant needling. Sometimes a trigger point has no effect. Many patients with a 'frozen shoulder' have a tender area over the insertion of the deltoid into the humerus. Needling this point never helps. It should be remembered that the needling of intramuscular trigger points, even for purely

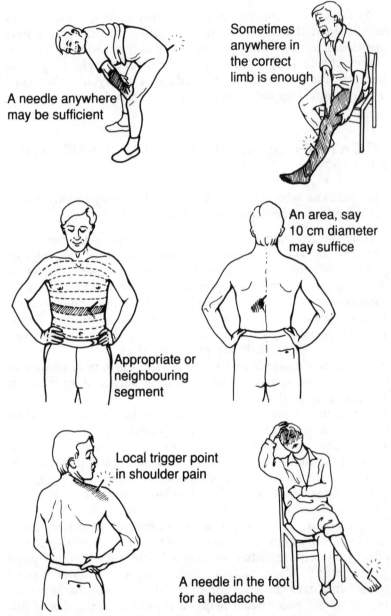

A needle anywhere may be sufficient

Sometimes anywhere in the correct limb is enough

An area, say 10 cm diameter may suffice

Appropriate or neighbouring segment

Local trigger point in shoulder pain

A needle in the foot for a headache

Fig. II.5

musculoskeletal problems, is only one aspect of acupuncture.

6 In traditional theory one can needle areas far removed from the site of symptoms, sometimes even at the opposite end of the body. This definitely works, though I think the areas which may be used are quite often different from those normally described and are effective for completely different reasons (Fig. II.5).

A consideration of the above six categories of acupuncture points, somewhat arbitrary though they may be, demonstrates that the classical idea of a very small acupuncture point in a fixed position is correct in relatively few instances.

At one time, when it was thought that acupuncture points were fixed in position, histologists tried to find something anatomically recognisable at acupuncture points. Some of them even 'succeeded' and published papers on the high concentration of specialised nerve endings at these points: motor end plates, neuromuscular spindles, neurotendinous spindles, the glomus arteriovenous anastomosis, organs of Golgi, Merkel's corpuscles, Vater–Pacini corpuscles, Meissner's corpuscles, terminal bulbs of Krause, free nerve ends, neurovascular bundles some 5 mm in diameter in the superficial fascia, etc. Others have tried to find changes in the electrical skin resistance at acupuncture points. However, my own experiments and the more exacting research of others (see my *Textbook of Acupuncture*, pp. 82–84) have failed to find evidence supporting any of these hypotheses.

As far as I am aware, nobody has even tried to find specialised nerve endings at McBurney's point, as it is obvious from its variable position that this could not occur. For me the same argument applies to the fruitless search for something that does not exist—the physical acupuncture point.

I do not know whether it is historically possible to discover the origins of Chinese acupuncture. The following might well be a possible scenario:

1 The early discoverers found certain tender areas of the body related to certain symptoms which, if stimulated, alleviated these symptoms, e.g. trigger points in the neck associated with shoulder pain. These tender areas are described in the earliest

extant Chinese sources in the vaguest of terms. To the best of my knowledge the ancient literature makes no definite statement about these areas, their size or shape or exact location; nor do the early drawings give an exact depiction, but only a vague indication.

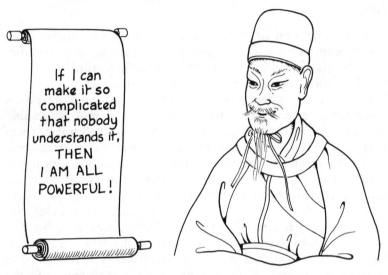

If I can make it so complicated that nobody understands it, THEN I AM ALL POWERFUL!

Fig. II.6 Possible thoughts of Chinese (and modern Western) scholars

2 At a later stage of the evolution of acupuncture, the Chinese scholars busied themselves with the subject. As is true of scholars the world over, they complicated the subject to render it worthy of a scholarly intellect (Fig. II.6). They added yin and yang, the five elements and other ideas of Taoist natural philosophy. They made it an exact knowledge with geometrically defined positions of acupuncture points.

3 Finally, when the West became aware of acupuncture the precise position of acupuncture points was already defined. Naturally the West imagined that this accuracy fitted in with the accuracy of a brain-child of the West, namely anatomy. Acupuncture points were no longer geometrically defined— they became anatomically defined.

This three-stage evolution is rather like a tale which, if it is repeated often enough, over several centuries, no longer resembles the original story. What I have tried to do is to base this book largely on original observations, not on acupuncture theory. I suspect that what I have written may well be similar to the reality underlying the earliest Chinese descriptions.

WHY SPECIFIC AREAS? AN UNSOLVED PROBLEM

If a patient has, say, appendicitis or toothache, he will have pain or tenderness or both in the abdomen or jaw, and possibly also in distant areas related to them. I presume, though I am not sure, that the threshold of stimulation at these painful or tender areas is lower than in normal areas of skin and subjacent tissue and thus a gentle pinprick is all that is required in treatment. In normal tissue the threshold of stimulation is higher and hence would require more massive stimulation to produce an effective treatment. The above mentioned 'facilitation' could occur at all levels of the nervous system (central, spinal, peripheral) and might in some instances involve a mechanism similar to the Gate Control Theory of Pain of Melzack and Wall, or the Diffuse Noxious Inhibitory Controls, utilising convergent neurones, of Le Bars, Besson and Dickenson. Many other neurological mechanisms might be involved, quite apart from neurochemical, neuroendocrine, chemical and other mechanisms. Further elucidation would be as useful for orthodox medicine as for acupuncture.

This raises a problem. Often one needles a distant area on the hand or foot to treat a disease of the abdomen, thorax or head. Usually these distant areas are not tender or painful and yet they are extremely effective, even with the gentlest of stimulation; indeed, my favourite acupuncture point, liver 3, between the 1st and 2nd metatarsals, is one such peripheral area. This I cannot explain unless one assumes that some sort of facilitation has taken place in lower centres of the brain or large sections of the spinal cord. A further field for research perhaps?

There are certain places in the body which are tender on pressure in the majority of people, of both sexes, whether or not they have any disease. Amongst them are: spleen 6, above the medial malleolus; spleen 9, below the knee medially; lung 5, over the head of the radius; and gall bladder 20, where the trapezius is attached to the occiput—all areas described in Part II of this book. These and other similarly tender areas are usually more effective in treatment than the normal 'acupuncture point' or area which only becomes tender in disease. I do not know why these permanently tender areas (provided they are related to the disease in question) are more effective than the areas which are only tender in disease—a still further field for research.

TYPE OF STIMULUS

In traditional acupuncture there are many different methods of stimulation, each of which is supposed to have a different effect: putting in a needle at right angles to the skin, or tangentially in the direction of the flow of Qi along a meridian or the very opposite; inserting the needle quickly and withdrawing it slowly, or the reverse; or using one, three, nine or 81 jabs; twisting the needle clockwise or anticlockwise. Sometimes these methods are combined and given such names as 'the green dragon wagging tail technique'. Sometimes, instead of a needle, heat is used in the form of moxa (the pith of artemisia), which may be burnt on the skin, in the air immediately above the skin or used to heat a needle. The skin may be slightly scarified with a 'plum flower needle', or bruised by cupping.

To all these the West has added modern technology, with electrical stimulation, laser beams and vibrators. At one time, due to a translation error, the majority of Western doctors differentiated between the effects of silver and gold acupuncture needles—something unknown in China. Some 'experts' even found a difference between needles made of stainless steel and molybdenum.

In my first few years in practice I diligently tried to differentiate between the effects of all the traditional methods mentioned above. When I started practising acupuncture, I believed in the tradition (nothing else was available) and hence of course wanted it to work. Despite this I found no difference between any of these methods.

Neither did I find any difference between needles made of silver, gold or stainless steel, though I have never tried molybdenum. I have tried electrical stimulation via surface electrodes and also with electrodes attached to subcutaneous or intramuscularly placed needles, again finding no particular difference. Some say there is a difference between slow stimulation (less than 10 Hz) and fast stimulation (over 100 Hz). This I have not investigated.

Lasers of various types are the latest state of the art. As no needle is involved, patients lose their fear of acupuncture. Moreover, there is no danger of hepatitis or acquired immune deficiency syndrome (AIDS). I have not tried a laser. Two of my colleagues, whose opinion I respect, Drs Alexander Macdonald and Douglas Golding, have tried them, the former with a neutral state of mind, whilst the latter was biased in favour of the laser working. Both found the effect of the laser to be less than that of the needle. The lasers used in acupuncture are weak. If they were stronger, as in 'star wars' films, I presume the effect would be greater! However, some doctors find lasers of particular benefit in children, who require gentle treatment. Others find they have an effect equal to needles in all patients, and a few find the effect greater than that of a needle. In this context it may be worth remembering that micro-acupuncture (see Chapter VII), which is a gentle form of acupuncture, may have a greater effect than periosteal acupuncture (see Part II), which stimulates strongly. Moreover, some patients are impressed by scientific-looking apparatus and therefore there could be an additional placebo effect (Fig. II.7).

I prefer using a disposable stainless steel needle, which I only leave in position for a few seconds. I feel I can control the 'dosage' more accurately with a hand-held needle than with an inanimate apparatus; not something I can prove scientifically, but real to me nevertheless. I feel that using one's hands in medicine is quite different from using machines: if my wife

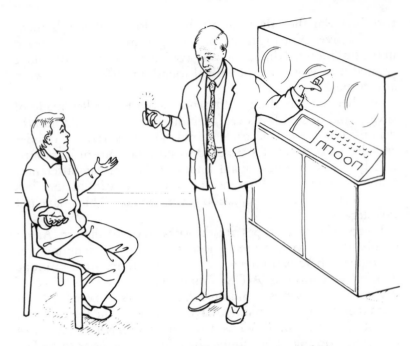

Fig. II.7 Doctor to patient: 'Would you like me to use this acupuncture needle worth 10 pence, or this scientific apparatus worth £1000?'

puts her hand on my thigh it has a different effect from a book placed on my thigh. Doctors will think this is purely psychological, though I think there is more to it. It should also be remembered that in many instances I needle the periosteum, which is easier to do with a needle than electrically or with a laser.

In my experience it does not matter what stimulus is used in acupuncture. I have little doubt that burning with a lighted cigarette, focusing the sun's rays with a magnifying glass, a drop of sulphuric acid or pinching the skin with a pair of pliers would all have the same effect as the more conventional stimuli used in acupuncture. All that is seemingly required is *to exceed the threshold of excitability*. Perhaps this is similar to nerve physiology which, as Adrian pointed out, responds in an 'all-or-none' manner (Fig. II.8).

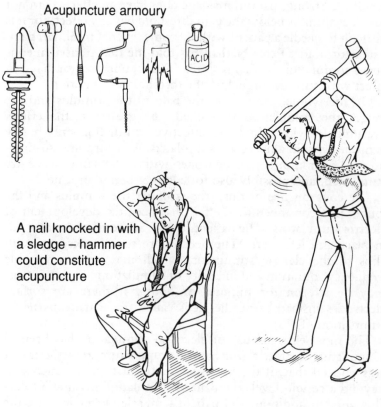

Acupuncture armoury

A nail knocked in with a sledge – hammer could constitute acupuncture

Fig. II.8

I once heard of a doctor who stimulated his patients so gently that instead of needling a specific place he would kiss it! I doubt if this would have breached the threshold of excitability, but I do not doubt it had some sort of effect on the patient!

STRENGTH OF STIMULUS

As mentioned above, it seems as if a certain threshold of excitability has to be exceeded before an effect can be achieved. Normal touch or, as mentioned previously, kissing, I think has no effect. Strong, painful massage does have an effect. I am not sure if a stimulus below the pain threshold has any effect, for it is difficult to needle a patient without some, even if minimal, pain. The neurologist Peter Nathan has told me that transcutaneous nerve stimulation, which is similar to acupuncture, can have an effect with stimulation below the threshold of sensation.

On the whole, the greater the pain of the stimulus and the longer the stimulation is applied, the greater is the effect. Presumably with minimally effective stimulation only a few neurones within a nerve are stimulated. With stronger stimulation a larger number of neurones within the same nerve are stimulated, and possibly also for a longer period of time.

The consequence of this, 'the stronger the stimulus and the longer it is continued the better', has been the development of electric stimulators. The patient has the appropriate needles put in place and left there. The needles are then hooked up with clips to the electric stimulator, which may have a variable frequency, duration and intensity of stimulation. The apparatus may be left on for minutes or hours. If there are surface electrodes instead of needles it is called transcutaneous nerve stimulation (TNS).

The most extreme use of electrical stimulation has been in acupuncture analgesia (misnamed acupuncture anaesthesia). It was noticed that, if the intensity of stimulation was increased beyond a certain level, the pain of stimulation became intolerable and, in addition, the patient's muscles went into tetanic spasm. To counteract this, the patient was given full premedication, lightly anaesthetised and curarised. In my opinion acupuncture analgesia is rarely of much use (see *Textbook of Acupuncture*, pp. 100–104).

The difficulty with 'the stronger the stimulus and the longer it is continued the better' is that not all patients respond to this sort of treatment. The reverse is true of some patients, namely 'the weaker the stimulus and the shorter time during which it is continued the better', described in Chapters IV and VII.

In traditional acupuncture the doctor puts the needle in place and then leaves it sticking in the patient for, say, 15 minutes. The ancients, who had no convenient watches, left the needle in for a certain number of breaths.

In my experience the needle only stimulates while it is manipulated and hurts a little, i.e. whilst piercing the skin, being twisted to and fro, pushed up and down, or pricking the periosteum—leaving it in place adds nothing. This may actually be observed in a certain type of patient.

A patient may have a pain which is alleviated within a few seconds of a single needle prick. The needle is then at once removed. The pain, however, returns, say 5 minutes later, when again a single pinprick will, within a few seconds, remove the pain for, again, 5 minutes. This procedure can be repeated several times, and on each occasion a few seconds of stimulation, followed by removal of the needle, produces freedom from pain for say 5 minutes.

If following this, or if the same patient is seen on a subsequent occasion, the same procedure is followed, except that after a few seconds' stimulation, the needle is not withdrawn but left in place, the result will be the same, namely some 5 minutes of freedom from pain. When the pain returns (the needle being *in situ*), the needle is given a few twists and again there is freedom from pain for some 5 minutes. This can be repeated *ad infinitum*. It is thus apparent that, whether the needle is left in place or not, it is only the stimulation which is effective. Sometimes, after needling, a patient may for a short while have a mild burning sensation around the needle insertion. This is the same, whether or not the needle is left in place.

It is for this reason that I do not leave needles in place. I think it is also less frightening for the patient, who no longer has to contend in his mind with the St Sebastian factor. Some patients may, however, benefit psychotherapeutically, as they think more is being done if the needles are left in place; in this case the longer they are left in place the better. There are a few doctors who use little needles, somewhat like drawing pins, which are left in place for about a week, covered with an adhesive dressing. This is supposed to be a form of continuous stimulation, I suppose a bit like TNS. I have never tried this method myself as I have seen patients who have had it done to them with results not much better, nor worse, than ordinary needling.

EXPERIMENTAL EVIDENCE THAT TRADITIONAL ACUPUNCTURE POINTS DO NOT EXIST

Most of the ideas expressed in this book are based on clinical experience, careful observation and questions. These observations, rather than research, have cast a doubt in my mind about whether classical acupuncture points really exist. Many will regard this as antediluvian, for today we have science.

Simple observation like mine has, for no apparent scientific reason, become unfashionable: most accepted research is done in laboratories. The days when the simple observations of Charles Darwin shook the world are past. However, I think acupuncture is different. At its present stage of development, it reveals its secrets more easily to quiet observation. It is such an elusive subject that it is extremely difficult even to know what to research. If so much is contradictory, what experiments does one do?

Despite what I have written above, orthodox medical research has its own, though different, part to play in trying to solve the enigma of acupuncture.

The first hundred pages of my *Textbook of Acupuncture* is devoted to a description of some fifty research projects in relation to acupuncture. The experiments show how stimulation of various parts of the surface may affect cardiac function, gastric tone, peristalsis, micturition, intestinal blood flow, movement of a distant limb, respiration, etc. in experimental animals. It was found in these experiments that there was an altered electrical activity in the sympathetic, parasympathetic or spinal innervation of the target area at the same time as the relevant part of the skin was stimulated, and that the above mentioned changes did not occur if the relevant nerve or nerve tract was divided. *All these 'reflexes' could be initiated by stimulating the body surface anywhere over quite a large area, i.e. the precision of an acupuncture point was not required.*

More recently Le Bars and colleagues* have recorded the

* Bing, Z., Villanueva, L. and Le Bars, D. Acupuncture-evoked responses of subnucleus reticularis dorsalis neurones in the rat medulla. *Neuroscience*, 1991, **44**: 693–703.

activity of the subnucleus reticularis dorsalis neurones in the rat medulla when stimulating an acupuncture point below the knee, called stomach 36, and comparing the effects with those obtained when stimulating a nearby non-acupuncture point. The result in both instances was the same.

All, or virtually all, neurophysiological research* on the distant effects of stimulating the skin show that the area of stimulus is a large one.

It is, of course, possible that all this experimental stimulation is only partially relevant to acupuncture, as these neurological effects normally only last for minutes, whereas the results of acupuncture may endure for days, weeks, months or years.

* See also the chapter on acupuncture by Alexander Macdonald in *Textbook of Pain* (eds P. D. Wall and R. Melzack), 1989, Churchill Livingstone, Edinburgh.

III

Radiation and the non-existent meridians

The so-called meridians are one of the most important features of traditional acupuncture. They supposedly explain the effect of needling the non-existent acupuncture points mentioned in the previous chapter.

The acupuncture meridians (a Western word) mimic, in some ways, the appearance of the meridians in geography, the majority being meridians of longitude rather than latitude (Fig. III.1). Depending on the method of counting, there are 12 or 20 or 59, which are described in detail in my *Textbook of Acupuncture* (pp. 305–468).

For years I have given many lectures to specialists in acupuncture, in which I have stated:

> 'The meridians of acupuncture are no more real than the meridians of geography. If someone were to get a spade and tried to dig up the Greenwich meridian, he might end up in a lunatic asylum. Perhaps the same fate should await those doctors who believe in meridians.'

The above provocative statement caused some doctors to close their ears; other doctors put me into the category of those unsavoury people who make tasteless jokes about a religion; still other doctors thought that perhaps I should go to the lunatic asylum. The only universal effect I achieved was to cause those who were dozing to wake up with a start. I was, I think, the first doctor to deny the existence of meridians, while at the same time offering a practical alternative, and I was

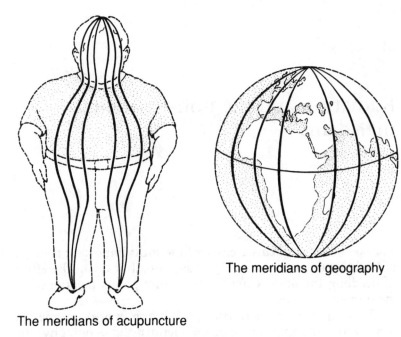

The meridians of geography

The meridians of acupuncture

Fig. III.1

greeted with the same incomprehension as when I denied the existence of acupuncture points. The remainder of this chapter will explain what I really mean.

RADIATION

If one needles certain parts of the body and, most particularly, if one needles the periosteum, the patient may feel a radiation.

If, for example, the periosteum of the sacro-iliac joint is needled there may be radiation down the leg. This radiation may (Fig. III.2):

1 Go down the back of the leg—perhaps slightly more often;
2 Go down the medial side of the leg;
3 Go down the lateral side of the leg;

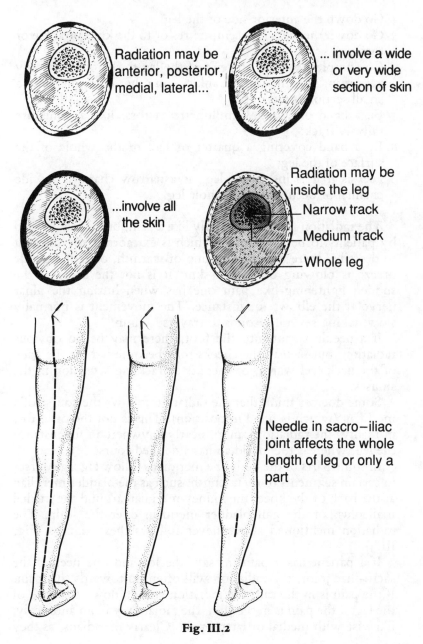

Radiation may be anterior, posterior, medial, lateral...

... involve a wide or very wide section of skin

...involve all the skin

Radiation may be inside the leg
Narrow track
Medium track
Whole leg

Needle in sacro-iliac joint affects the whole length of leg or only a part

Fig. III.2

33

4 Go down the anterior side of the leg;
5 Go down the leg a few centimetres or to the knee or ankle or toes;
6 Go completely from one end of the leg to the other or only appear in, say, the shin or ankle—on other occasions only a small section is left out;
7 Be a band only a few millimetres across, like a miniature railway track;
8 Be a band covering a quarter or half or the whole of the surface of the leg;
9 Feel as if it is inside the leg, as a narrow channel, a wide channel or occupying the whole leg.

The radiation feels occasionally like a pain, but is usually said by patients to be a sensation which is extraordinarily difficult to describe: there may be a feeling of warmth, or as if a gentle breeze is blowing on to the skin. It is not the same as the sudden lightening-like pain one has when hitting the ulnar nerve at the elbow, for instance. The movement is normally slow, taking several seconds to traverse a limb.

If a needle is put into the foot, there may be no obvious radiation, but instead the cheeks may become red, or the back of the neck feel warm, or there is a crackling sensation in the sinuses.

Some doctors think that the radiation follows the course of a meridian (which is fixed in position). This is not the case, for, in reality, the radiation can go nearly anywhere in for instance the leg, whereas the meridian has a defined course.

In some parts of the body the meridians follow zigzag courses in certain segments of their length, such as the bladder meridian at the back of the knee, the kidney meridian around the medial malleolus, or the gall bladder meridian over the scalp. The radiation mentioned above never follows these zigzags (Fig. III.3).

If a patient has a pain in, say, the leg and one needles the sacro-iliac joint, the radiation will often go towards this pain. If the pain is in the calf, the radiation will go down the back of the leg; if the pain is in the shin, the radiation will go anteriorly; likewise with medial or lateral pain. Clearly meridians, as they

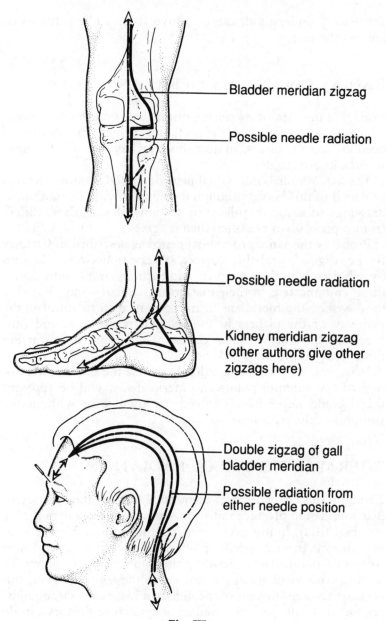

Bladder meridian zigzag

Possible needle radiation

Possible needle radiation

Kidney meridian zigzag
(other authors give other
zigzags here)

Double zigzag of gall
bladder meridian

Possible radiation from
either needle position

Fig. III.3

are usually understood, cannot move around like columns of
ants on the march.

RADIATION VERSUS MERIDIANS

I imagine the idea of meridians originated with the prehistoric
Chinese, who observed the radiation which can occur on
needling specific places. In time this may have become the rigid
scheme known to us.

The actual radiation that happens described in most sections
of Part II of this book, although it coincides with the traditional
drawings of some meridians or sections of meridians, differs
from it probably more often than it agrees.

Probably the same process happened as described in Chapter
II: the original, probably correct, observations were taken up
by scholars who then processed something simple into something complicated, in their masterful, scholarly way. Possibly
they wished the meridians in microcosm man to simulate the
pathway of the planets in the celestial macrocosm and thus
produced the truly amazing course of the meridians, coursing
three times round the whole body.

However, despite the fact that I criticise the present description of acupuncture points and meridians, it will be apparent
that I could never have evolved my own ideas without the
stimulus of the traditional structures.

THERAPEUTIC USE OF RADIATION

Earlier in this chapter it was mentioned that needling the sacro-
iliac joint could produce radiation virtually anywhere in the leg
(see Fig. III.2). In my experience, conditions found in the areas
of radiation from a specific point are susceptible to treatment
from that point. Thus, needling the joint could, in theory, be
used to treat virtually any condition in the leg. However, this
is rather too reminiscent of the indiscriminate use of tranquillisers for 'difficult' patients. Skilled acupuncture doctors can do
better.

Needling the sacro-iliac joint may, under certain circumstances, be the best treatment, as in some cases of sciatica. In other instances a completely different treatment may be more appropriate. It often requires considerable skill to decide which is the best treatment. If, for example, the patient has a pain in the knee, a more effective treatment might be to needle a tender area just below the medial condyle of the tibia. It must, however, be said that needling the sacro-iliac joint may have a slight effect and, on rare occasions, even be the best treatment.

If the anterior aspect of the head of the radius, or capitulum of the humerus, is needled, the commonest radiation is down the lateral side of the arm to the thumb, and hence a pain in the thumb may be treated in this way (Fig. III.4). The radiation

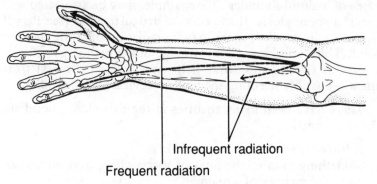

Infrequent radiation

Frequent radiation

Fig. III.4 Needle head of radius anteriorly, or capitulum

from the head of the radius may, rarely, go to the medial side of the lower arm and also to the little finger, though, as this is rare, it is likewise rarely of much use in treating disease of the 5th finger. If the patient has pain at the base of the thumb, in the 1st carpometacarpal joint, needling the anterior side of the base of the 1st metacarpal is often more effective than needling the head of the radius, though it may be preferable to needle the head of the radius as a first attempt as it is less painful and less likely to cause a reaction.

A detailed description of the radiation that may be experienced when needling the periosteum is given in Part II of this book. This may afford the doctor preliminary indications of possible methods of treatment, which, however, may or may not be the most appropriate in any individual case.

It should be remembered that the possible variations in radiation are infinite and therefore some variations have not been described or illustrated. There are two factors which help selection:

1 A knowledge of which radiation is more common or less common. If the symptoms of the patient coincide with a common pattern of radiation, the treatment is more likely to be effective than if they coincide with a less common pattern of radiation.

2 A knowledge of medicine in general. Some of the milder cases of 'painful shoulder', for example, may be associated with cervical spondylosis. If the cervical articular pillar (see Part II, Section 4) is needled, there may be radiation over the shoulder joint. Thus, combining a knowledge of the pathology with the course of the radiation may help one to select the best treatment—possibly needling the tender cervical articular pillar.

There have been many theories in the past about meridians; these included:

A force emanating from the chakras.
Something akin to the lines of force which iron filings take up in the vicinity of a magnet.
The course of nerves, arteries, veins or lymphatics.

I once had a theory comparing the meridians to the lateral line system in fish, which is more extensive than normally illustrated. This was published in the 1962 edition of my *Acupuncture: The Ancient Chinese Art of Healing*. I quickly discarded this theory.

This chapter, which describes what I have thought for over 25 years, is my present contribution. I have, however, little idea what the cause of the radiation might be, though I suspect it is the barely recognised sympathetic and parasympathetic afferents (not efferents) whose effects are modified by spinal and higher centres.

Radiation occurs more frequently and over a considerably

greater distance in Strong Reactors (see Chapter IV). The more radiation occurs, the more likely it is that a specific treatment will be effective.

IV

Strong Reactors
Strong Reactors and drugs

Within a few weeks of starting my own practice in acupuncture in 1959, I realised that there were basically two types of patient:

1 *Strong reactors* These patients respond to acupuncture like magic. Their symptoms may be cured or alleviated within seconds or minutes of treatment, a treatment which involves only one or two needles and gentle stimulation.
2 *Normal reactors* These patients are the normal, plodding, foot soldiers. Their symptoms may improve only several days after treatment, or even only after several treatments. The treatment requires more needles and stronger stimulation.

Most of this chapter is devoted to these Strong Reactors, who form perhaps a third of the population, who require much gentler treatment by acupuncture and who possibly form a substantial proportion of the patients who have 'adverse reactions' to normal dosages of drugs. I am proud to have discovered something which was hardly mentioned in the ancient literature and yet is of the greatest importance to successful practice. It is possibly just as important to doctors practising orthodox medicine and to the drug industry.

STRONG REACTORS AND HYPER-STRONG REACTORS

1 *Results* As mentioned above, Strong Reactors are cured amazingly rapidly. Sometimes within seconds or minutes of perhaps a single subcutaneous needle prick, left in place for a few seconds, these patients may be cured or have a reduction in symptoms of an illness which they have had for days, weeks, months or even years.

A few minutes after treatment, I may ask such patients if their headache has gone, if they can turn their neck, if they can raise their legs or touch their toes, or whatever I need to know to ascertain the result of treatment. Often the patients hesitate, thinking they have misheard my question, for after all, every sensible person knows that medicine cannot work so quickly. I then reassure the patients that they have not misheard me (I sometimes have a quiet voice), and would they please answer my question. It then gives me the greatest pleasure, not to listen, but just to watch the patient's expression of stunned disbelief, features paralysed with incredulity. They feel or have observed the impossible, they just do not know how to think or react, for they have observed a 'miracle'; they are cured, or there is at least a substantial amelioration of their symptoms. Sometimes the devout mention passages from the Bible or make comparisons with Lourdes.

Unfortunately, the above experience does not happen every day, but I am sure that most experienced doctors who practice acupuncture have noticed it occasionally. With the correct technique, described in this chapter, it can happen more often. It should be remembered though that the really dramatic responses to acupuncture, those that seem miraculous, happen not in the ordinary Strong Reactors, but rather in what might be called the Hyper-Strong Reactors, who form, possibly, 5% of the population (Fig. IV.1).

2 *Strength of treatment* The type of response described above occurring in a Hyper-Strong Reactor, or the lesser versions of it occurring daily in ordinary Strong Reactors, is an indication that the patient requires gentle treatment.

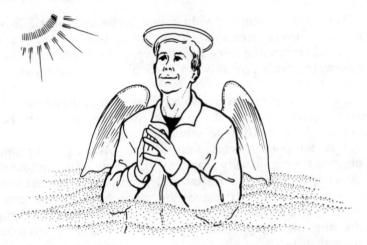

Fig. IV.1 A Hyper-Strong Reactor may feel he is in heaven after acupuncture

In the most responsive patients a single, subcutaneous or intracutaneous prick with a thin needle, left in place for a few seconds, is sufficient. On very rare occasions, only one treatment is required. My aim, rarely realised, is to cure most patients with one needle prick in one treatment.

Somewhat stronger treatments are required in the majority of patients. The strength of treatment may be increased by:

(a) Twisting the needle to and fro, pushing it up and down, or other painful manoeuvres.

(b) Instead of using a smoothly polished needle, using one with a rougher surface.

(c) Using a needle whose tip is less finely tapered, or of larger diameter.

(d) Deeper needling.

(e) Periosteal acupuncture. Strong Reactors require only one slight touch of the periosteum to achieve an immediate response, such as radiation, a warm feeling, blushing or relief of symptoms.

(f) Needling a larger number of places.

(g) Performing a larger number of treatments.

There is no distinct dividing line between Normal Reactors and Strong Reactors. It is rather like the height of people: there are the very tall, the very short and everything in between, with probably no particular accentuation of any particular region.

3 *Results of over-treatment* also *signs of effective treatment* If a Strong Reactor is treated too strongly there may easily be a reaction, the symptoms of which are often:

(a) A temporary worsening of the patient's symptoms. This worsening usually happens the same evening or the following morning. If, for example, the patient, suffers from migraine and is overtreated, he may have an extremely severe migraine the same evening or following morning. This migraine may be of the usual duration or even last longer than usual.

This reaction may be unpleasant or even extremely unpleasant, but it is never permanent. In drug therapy, patients sometimes have adverse reactions which, if the drug is stopped at once, normally abate. In a few instances, however, the adverse reactions to drugs are permanent. This does not happen in acupuncture.

I imagine that the reactions to acupuncture are temporary because acupuncture is essentially such a gentle treatment, best suited to the correction of easily reversible physiological processes such as migraine. Drugs, generally speaking, exert a more powerful influence and are often used to treat diseases which are much more than 'easily reversible physiological processes', such as congestive cardiac failure, pneumonia, etc., where acupuncture is of little use.

In a few instances, a doctor practising acupuncture should tread with caution. If an asthmatic, for example, were to have a reaction to treatment, he might develop status asthmaticus and require immediate hospitalisation. It is, therefore, advisable to treat asthmatics extremely gently on the first one or two occasions, until one is able to judge with certainty how they respond.

Case history. A patient had had headaches on most days for several years. I judged that he had the 'liver' type of headache and treated his liver at liver 3 (dorsalis pedis/dorsal interosseous area) in the normal way. Nothing happened while he was in my consulting room, but that same evening he developed a headache which was severe and lasted longer than usual.

The next time I saw him, 2 weeks later, I made sure that my wife (herself a Hyper-Strong Reactor and thus alive to it in others) opened the door to him. She thought he was one of those, not so obvious, Strong Reactors. Therefore on the second occasion I did not treat him normally, as I had done on the first occasion, but instead treated him with the strength of needling suitable for a 1-year-old baby, using the same place on the foot. Immediately after treatment he felt relaxed, and from then onwards his headaches started improving, until finally he was about 80% cured.

(b) Strong Reactors often feel relaxed or even sleepy after treatment; some actually fall asleep. I frequently have patients who doze or sleep in my consulting rooms for anything from 30 minutes to even 4 hours. Some feel tired on the way home and would like to lie down and sleep on the pavement (Fig. IV.2). These are all good signs and show that the treatment is working well. If a patient has this type of response, the treatment is more likely to work.

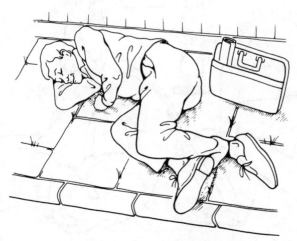

Fig. IV.2 If on the way home the patient lies down on the pavement to go to sleep, he has been overtreated

Sometimes, however, a patient feels sleepy for a week afterwards, or he may feel lethargic and knocked out. In this instance the treatment has been too strong and should, on the subsequent occasion, be gentler.

(c) Sometimes after treatment, particularly in Strong Reactors, patients become euphoric and overenergetic, though this is less frequent than the relaxation and sleepiness mentioned under (b). These patients may go home and mow the lawn and even their neighbour's lawn. They may start spring-cleaning the house and continue nearly non-stop until it is finished (Fig. IV.3). A patient might keep his wife awake all night (illustration censored), but it does not last. There are also a few patients who are relaxed, perhaps even a little sleepy, but euphoric at the same time.

I have had a few patients who have been drug addicts in a minor way or who, on rare occasions, smoked a 'joint'.

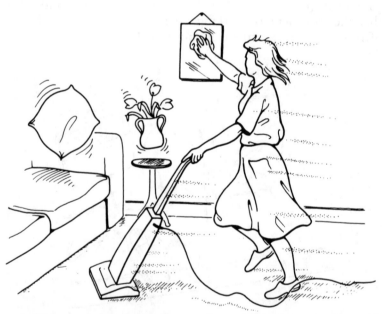

Fig. IV.3 If a patient starts spring-cleaning their house immediately after acupuncture, they have been struck by the euphoric effect of acupuncture

They have told me that the 'high' obtained with drugs is similar to that obtained by acupuncture, though that obtained by acupuncture is more erratic and less strong.

A very few patients laugh uncontrollably after acupuncture, for a few minutes or even for several hours. Whatever one tells them—sad, funny or factual—or even if one just sits in silence, the laughter bubbles up like water from a spring.

There are also a few who laugh and cry alternately for a few minutes at a time.

In (b) above I described the Strong Reactor who felt relaxed and sleepy after treatment, which is a good sign in moderation, though if it continues for a week it is a sign of overtreatment, which should on subsequent occasions be gentler. In (c) I have described the Strong Reactors who become overenergetic or euphoric. This is always a good sign and is an indication that the treatment is more likely to succeed. I have never met a patient where this signified overtreatment.

If a patient has a reaction, I normally think it best to do nothing and ask the patient to wait a few hours or days until the reaction automatically wears off. If, which is rare, the reaction is excessive, one can do the following: if the patient has migraine and overtreatment at liver 3 (dorsalis pedis/dorsal interosseous area) gave him a severe long-lasting attack, then the same place, liver 3, can be needled *extremely gently*, as if the patient were a 6-month-old baby. Usually the migraine will then abate, sometimes even within minutes.

RADIATION AND STRONG REACTORS

Strong Reactors have radiation much more frequently than Normal Reactors.

If a needle is inserted into a Normal Reactor intradermally, subcutaneously or intramuscularly, the patient usually has a little pain at the site of insertion, which may form an area of pain around the needle a few centimetres in diameter. Occasionally there is radiation extending for 5 or 10 cm, as described in Chapter III. If a small nerve is hit inadvertently, there is, of course, a different type of sensation—a shooting pain.

In traditional acupuncture, once the needle is in place one tries to manipulate it to produce radiation, as it is well known that, if one has radiation, the resultant treatment is usually better. This manipulation is achieved by twisting the needle to and fro, pushing it up and down, and by slightly altering its position. The latter can be done by completely reinserting the needle or by leaving the needle in the skin and angling the tip in different directions. After all this manipulation, which can be quite painful and entails the risk of overtreatment, radiation is achieved in some patients.

In Strong Reactors, just needling the correct, often tender, point often produces radiation to a greater or lesser extent. The radiation may extend only 10 cm, or it may extend from one end of the body to the other.

In a Strong Reactor there may be not the normal type of radiation, but instead a reddening of the cheeks, warmth at the back of the neck, a general warmth or feeling of relaxation, responses which are described in Chapter III.

In most Chinese books it is recognised that the achievement of radiation signifies a greater chance of successful treatment. This is usually ascribed to the correct manipulation of the needle in the correct place. I think this is rarely the case, but is usually due to needling a Strong Reactor.

At one time I tried needling peripheral nerves as I hoped I might achieve better results than with normal needling. As anaesthetists and pain specialists know, the needling of a peripheral nerve produces a sharp lightning-like pain which goes peripherally, quite unlike the slow-moving sensation, which is rarely pain, of radiation. I noticed that this lightning pain was achieved more easily, with less manipulation of the needle, in Strong Reactors. Presumably the diameter of peripheral nerves in Strong Reactors and Normal Reactors is the same, but perhaps the threshold of stimulation in the Strong Reactor is lower.

STRONG REACTORS AND DRUGS

In a practice solely devoted to acupuncture, such as mine, it is of course very common to see some patients who come because they are disenchanted with orthodox medicine, much as I see occasional Christian Scientists (who are not supposed to see doctors) as, perversely, they think I am not a real doctor. Nevertheless, if I were the only doctor in a small village (instead of one of many in the specialist district of Central London), I would practise orthodox medicine much of my time, for there are innumerable diseases where orthodox drugs *in the correct dose* are the best treatment. Why should I be against orthodox medicine when it once saved my life?

The reason that some patients come to me or, for that matter, to doctors practising other forms of alternative medicine, is because they or their relatives have experienced adverse reactions with drugs. Many such patients just feel more ill with their medicines than without! Some feel so ill for months on end that they think they are slowly dying, until they stop their drugs or change them. I have seen patients who have permanently acquired purple/brown nails, lost their hair only to see it regrow in a different colour like that of a golliwog, have collapsed vertebrae . . . the list is endless, known to all doctors, and well described in, for example, the British National Formulary.

Many of these adverse reactions could be avoided . . .

Specific patients who often react badly to drugs

I ask most patients how they react to drugs, for it is an indication as to who might or might not be a Strong Reactor to acupuncture.

1 There are many patients who take whatever their doctors prescribe. The medicine works as well as might be expected and there are infrequent adverse reactions. These patients usually do not feel ill or in any way peculiar while taking their medicine. Mostly, but by no means always, these patients are,

from an acupuncture point of view, Normal Reactors, the type of patient most orthodox doctors prefer, for without much thought one can prescribe a standard drug and a standard dose. These patients may have adverse reactions on rare occasions, but the essential characteristic of this group is that they are rare.

2 There are other patients, a substantial minority, whose response to drugs is different:

(a) They respond normally to drugs on most occasions, but the side-effects are a little more frequent than one might hope.

(b) The side-effects occur moderately frequently, very frequently, or nearly always.

(c) Some more adventurous or intelligent patients may have discovered that if they take a smaller dose than prescribed, their medicine works perfectly well, with the added bonus of no side-effects. There are not many such patients, for most accept blindly what their doctor says, or else reject his advice altogether and take no drugs whatsoever.

All the patients in group (2) are probably, but not necessarily, Strong Reactors.

Treatment of Strong Reactors

Strong Reactors are difficult to treat. A specific patient may need:

Three-quarters of the normal dose of drug A.
Half the normal dose of drug B.
A quarter of the normal dose of drug C.
A tenth of the normal dose of drug D.
The normal dose of drug E.
And, rarely, double the normal dose of drug F.

All these different responses to drugs A–F can happen in one single patient. This single patient may respond as a Normal Reactor to say aspirin or paracetamol, but will require, say, a quarter of the normal dose of a tranquilliser. If this patient takes the reduced dose the drug works well, with few or no side-effects.

There are a few Strong Reactors who are not as variable as mentioned above. These require, say, three-quarters of the normal dose of nearly all drugs or, if they are more sensitive, all drug dosages can be halved.

It is extraordinarily difficult for a doctor to know what is best under these circumstances. The most important thing, however, is to know that these people exist and that they form a substantial minority. Apart from this, the doctor needs time, the ability and willingness to listen and an open mind.

There are some patients, at least in my practice, who have never taken a drug and hence one cannot ask them about the way they have responded in the past to their various medicines. Some of this group will display a mild subconscious fear of drugs: they just have the feeling that, at least for them, drugs are not the right answer. They have no logical reason for this attitude; it is perhaps a type of instinct. Repeated experience in my practice has shown that this instinct is usually correct and that these patients are Strong Reactors.

I have the impression from my practice that the majority of the side-effects of drugs, particularly if they are not too severe, are not mentioned by the patient to their general practitioner, as they know from previous experience that it arouses little interest, or 'you have to balance the benefit against the adverse reaction'.

I am sure that the commonest cause for both mild and severe adverse reactions is due to the prescription of the wrong dose to Strong Reactors. If this were more generally recognised, orthodox drug-based medicine would lose some of its dangers and become (to put it in modern parlance) more 'user friendly'. It is said, though I do not know if it is true, that a third of disease is iatrogenic. Part of this one-third would thus be avoided. Patients would also appreciate their doctors more, for they would notice they were being treated as individuals and not merely as standard, average penny-in-the-slot machines. Some drugs, whose use has been forbidden or whose manufacture has even been stopped, might still be in use today if it had been recognised who is and who is not a Strong Reactor. That said, there may, of course, be some drugs that are toxic for everyone, Strong Reactor and Normal Reactor alike.

The great difficulty with Strong Reactors is to know what dose to give them. Should one start with three-quarters of the normal dose or one-tenth of the normal dose? In a chronic disease one can usually start with a very low dose. If there is no effect, the dose can be increased gradually until there is a therapeutic effect or the earliest beginnings of side-effects. If the side-effects appear first, another drug can be tried instead, with which one hopes that the therapeutic effect occurs at a lower dosage than the side-effect.

Acute emergencies, however, are a different ball game and there I see no easy solutions. However, I think my contribution to orthodox drug-based medicine will be as great as that to acupuncture if this idea of Strong Reactors and drugs becomes part of accepted medical wisdom.

HOW TO DIAGNOSE A STRONG REACTOR

To know who is or who is not a Strong Reactor, or to gauge who is a Hyper-Strong Reactor, is extraordinarily difficult. You cannot send a test off to the laboratory. You have to find out yourself.

There are many indications; the first mentioned below is the most reliable and yet the most difficult.

1 One has the impression that the Strong Reactor has a body and mind which has not been cast in a rigid, immutable mould. If one were to imagine a human-being as consisting of a hundred parts then, in the Normal Reactor, these hundred parts are joined together with glue and are immobile, whereas in a Strong Reactor the hundred parts are lubricated with oil and can easily be moved around.

In a certain way Strong Reactors are more sensitive; they may be able to feel somebody looking at them from behind; they are more intuitive, knowing for no real reason what has happened in the past or may happen in the future. A Strong Reactor can look at the setting sun and be quite overcome, and even shattered at its beauty, whilst a Normal Reactor just sees a red blob on the horizon and might think about which way the light is refracted.

Being a Strong Reactor or Normal Reactor has nothing to do with a neurotic tendency or phlegmatic tendency; being thin or fat; being tall or short; being clever, intelligent or dumb; being male or female, young or old; being physically sturdy or a weakling; being well educated or poorly educated; having a skin which is white, black, yellow or brown; having finely chiselled features or coarse features; being honest or a liar; being rich or poor; belonging to the nobility or being a peasant.

One can sometimes tell from the tone of a patient's voice on the telephone whether he is likely to be a Strong Reactor. What is actually said or the choice of words is less important. It is rather the tone and manner of speech which give an indication.

My impression is that a Strong Reactor belongs to a certain *physiological* type. It is neither a purely *physical* nor a purely *mental* characteristic. A Strong Reactor just functions in a certain way, much as an Eskimo can digest blubber, whilst most of us cannot.

2 Strong Reactors often react differently to drugs, usually requiring a smaller than average dose and having more frequent adverse reactions, as mentioned in detail in the previous section on Strong Reactors and Drugs. This drug idiosyncrasy, however, is far from universal, occurring in perhaps only half the Strong Reactors.

3 Strong Reactors respond better to, but also more frequently have a 'reaction' to acupuncture, i.e. a temporary worsening of symptoms.

They respond to gentler treatment.

They more frequently have radiation or other distant effects.

They feel relaxed, fall asleep or become euphoric more easily.

All these effects, discussed earlier in this chapter, can only be ascertained *after* treatment. It is better to know *before* treatment, as described in (1) and (2) above.

4 Rarely, particularly with a Hyper-Strong Reactor, I have the feeling as if 'electricity' is passing between the patient and myself. It is similar to that *je ne sais quoi* that passes between lovers even when they are not touching one another. It is a sort of electrified atmosphere. It has nothing to do with sex, occurring in patients of either gender.

5 It might perhaps be of interest to describe my wife's approach

to recognising Strong Reactors. Her method—in so far as anything so insubstantial and evanescent can be called a method—has evolved, in the 5 years or so that she has been concerned with the reactor status of patients, from a purely personal and irrational empathy with fellow Strong Reactors— using her 'nose' as it were—to a more systematic approach which is both communicable to others and can also be used by those who are not themselves Strong Reactors. All that is necessary is the capacity to observe people and a good mental filing system.

Once a patient has been treated a few times, or sometimes even after only one treatment, we know from experience how strongly he reacts. Moreover, Strong Reactors do often have a kind of psychosomatic resemblance to other Strong Reactors. Resemblance is actually too strong a word: I use it for want of a better one. It is an impression as insubstantial and delicate as a butterfly's wing, rather as one can catch a fleeting likeness between two very distantly related people who do not obviously resemble one another. This does not mean that all Strong Reactors resemble all other Strong Reactors: that would be too easy! There are as many degrees and ways of being a Strong Reactor as there are people. However, where this frail likeness exists between one patient and another treated some time previously, the former will turn out to be a Strong Reactor in the same way and approximately to the same degree as the latter, earlier patient. The stronger the 'family' resemblance, the more similar the reactor status.

With time and experience one can build up an extensive mental cross-reference system. My wife has a mental picture of it as an iridescent cobweb of delicate threads running from patient to patient. More mundanely, she finds this the easiest and most accurate way of assessing whether and to what degree a certain patient is a Strong Reactor.

GENERALITIES

It is thus apparent that being a Strong Reactor involves the whole person. We are on a different, more holistic plane from the more usual classification of body types.

As far as I am aware, the disease which patients have has little effect on their reactor status. It might be imagined that those suffering from allergic diseases are more likely to be Strong Reactors, but I think that this is not the case. The sole exception is patients with ME (myalgic encephalomyelitis or postviral fatigue). I have seen over 30 such patients and all responded as Strong Reactors. Whether they were already Strong Reactors before they became ill or only as a result of the illness is difficult to know, though I have the strong impression they have been Strong Reactors since birth. I likewise have the impression, but in this instance I am far less sure, that patients with multiple sclerosis are also Strong Reactors.

The diagnosis of Strong Reactors is an art, it is not a science. I do not think it will ever be a science. I do not belong to the school which thinks that one day everything in the universe will be explained by science, for then, to my way of thinking, we would be little more than intelligent computers.

Formerly I used to think that perhaps 10–30% of the population were Strong Reactors. However, when I married, my wife, being a Strong Reactor, was often able to recognise them better than I could, for she felt a certain empathy with other Strong Reactors. As a result we recognised that an ever-increasing proportion of patients were Strong Reactors and, at the moment, we think it is 50%, or nearly 50% of patients. Whether this high figure of 50% would apply to the population in general I do not know, for perhaps such patients are either subconsciously attracted to me, because I understand the problems associated with being a Strong Reactor, or are more likely to come to a practice such as this because they have had unfortunate experiences with orthodox medicine.

It is commonly thought that one cannot have too much of a good thing. Hence many doctors think they will achieve better results with their patients with stronger stimulation. Thus they put many needles in their patients, using needles which are both thick and long, perhaps reinforced with 30 minutes' electrostimulation, the whole process reminiscent of the martyrdom of St Sebastian. I occasionally see these abundantly punctured patients who have not been cured (those that are cured I do not see). Instead, if I recognise that they are Strong

Reactors, I may place one thin needle for a few seconds in their skin, with a resultant immediate improvement in some of them—others are still failures. I cannot give a scientific explanation for this except that I recognise that a gentle kiss may have a greater effect than a tough kiss, or that a gentle waft of perfume may attract, whereas a strong one repels (Fig. IV.4).

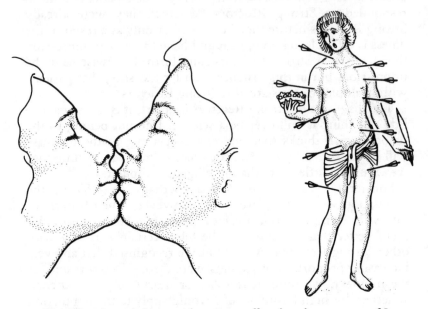

Fig. IV.4 A gentle kiss may have more effect than the treatment of St Sebastian

A few years ago I was reading an English translation by Ki Sunu of what is probably the oldest Chinese medical book, the *Huangti Nei Ching Ling Shu.*★ In it there is a chapter on the Physical Constitution of the Fat and Lean Person. It consists of a description of the Fat Type, who should be needled strongly, and the Lean Type, who should be needled gently.

The Fat Type is a strong, young man, who moves slowly, is fat, has a big body, wide shoulders, thick lower lip and dark skin and flesh. Elsewhere I read that he belonged to the labouring, peasant class.

The Lean Type is weak, lean, has thin skin and flesh, moves quickly, has a poor complexion, thin lips and a white colour. Elsewhere I read that he belonged to the scholarly class or nobility.

Clearly the above description is vastly different from that of the Normal Reactor and of the Strong Reactor. In my experience it is not usually the case that 'strong, thickset peasants' need strong treatment, or that 'weak, thin scholars' need gentle treatment. Alas, the difference between Normal and Strong Reactors is neither so obvious nor so clear-cut. It is evident that the ancient Chinese realised there was a difference between the two groups, but the text describes the differences one possibly might suppose to exist—practical reality being rather different. Perhaps the text was partially falsified on purpose so that undesirable people would not know the secret of success, a practice which was extensive in medieval Europe and might not have been unknown in China.

It is apparent from this chapter that a description of Strong Reactors is extraordinarily difficult, and hence it could have eluded verbal definition. Perhaps there do exist old books with a more accurate description, of which I am unaware; however, the concept of Strong Reactors and Normal Reactors is certainly not a part of the everyday normal practice of acupuncture in China today.

* *The Canon of Acupuncture*, Vol. I, pp. 330–331. Translated by Ki Sunu, 1985, Yuin University Press, Los Angeles.

V

The liver or upper digestive dysfunction

A colleague, or should I write 'anti-colleague', has on several occasions said: 'Felix Mann knows nothing about acupuncture apart from liver 3.' France, as is well known, is the centre of the world in matters pertaining to the liver, so this gentleman, being a Frenchman, should have known better.

In Anglo-Saxon countries the word *liver* signifies the actual anatomical liver, and hence is associated with diseases such as cirrhosis, jaundice, hepatitis, hepatic tumours, etc. As a young doctor I worked for 6 months in Strasbourg in eastern France and became acquainted with quite a different concept of the *liver*. It is a concept used more by doctors practising unortho-dox medicine and by the laity than by the high priests of the orthodox. The traditional Chinese concept of the liver (see *Textbook of Acupuncture*, pp. 395–403) is likewise different from both the French general usage and Western medical ideas.

I have taken the French and Chinese ideas and transfused them with my experience of acupuncture. My logical mind has dictated that *if it works and, on repeated occasions, the patients feel better, the theory is at least a practical working hypothesis.* My experience fits in largely, but far from completely, with that of the French. I should add that this French idea is fairly well diffused in most of Southern Europe and, I believe, to some extent in Eastern Europe and North Africa, particularly amongst the practitioners and patients of indigenous medical systems.

Those of you who read further will become aware that what is called, by the French and myself, 'being livery' does not concern only the *liver*, but is really a *dysfunction of all or several of the upper abdominal organs: the liver, gall bladder, digestive function of the pancreas, stomach, duodenum and probably the jejunum.* In some instances there may be a dysfunction of all these organs, whereas in other instances the dysfunction may affect mainly one or two organs. Perhaps I should no longer use the word liver and instead adopt the phrase *upper digestive dysfunction.* Usually I use both expressions, but mainly the word liver, for this is normal usage in France and elsewhere, the context clarifying which type of liver is alluded to.

Innervation

The innervation of all the upper abdominal organs is nearly identical:

The sympathetic innervation is via the coeliac ganglion, which receives fibres from the greater and lesser splanchnic nerves whose origin is from T5 to T12.* The liver also has an innervation via nerves carried in the peritoneal folds, presumably from the same segments.

The parasympathetic innervation is via the vagus, which carries fibres to and from the medulla.

According to the well-known book of Hansen and Schliack,* the innervation of the upper abdominal organs based on the clinical observation of areas of muscle tension, vasomotor phenomena, piloerection, superficial and deep tenderness, is as follows:

Liver and gall bladder	T6 to T10	sometimes T5 to T12
Pancreas	T7 to T9	
Stomach	T5 to T9	sometimes T4 to L1
Duodenum	T6 to T10	
Jejunum	T8 to T11	

* *Gray's Anatomy*, Longman, London.
* Hansen, K. and Schliak, H. *Segmentale Innervation. Ihre Bedeutung für Klinik und Praxis*, Georg Thieme, Stuttgart.

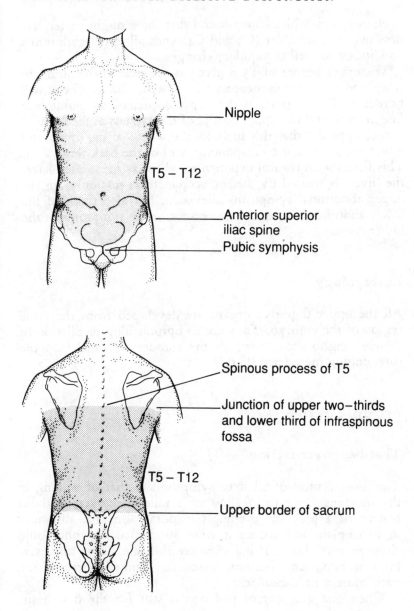

Fig. V.1

Hansen and Schliack also found that there might be tenderness over the shoulder (C3 and C4) with all upper abdominal conditions, as well as pupillary changes.

The upper border of T5 is given as the level of the nipple in front and the spinous process of T5 at the back. The lower border of T12 is given as the upper border of the pubic hair line in front and the upper border of the sacrum at the back. It is thus apparent that this includes the whole of the upper and lower abdomen and corresponding area of the back (Fig. V.1). This fits in with clinical experience: when, as mentioned later, the 'liver' is treated by diet or acupuncture, not only are the upper abdominal symptoms alleviated, but also those of the lower abdomen and, to a lesser extent, some symptoms in the lower chest.

Embryology

All the upper digestive organs are developed from the same region of the embryo. They are an outpouching or dilation of closely neighbouring parts of the entodermal canal into the surrounding mesoderm (Fig. V.2*).

LIVER SYMPTOMS

That hangover feeling

The most typical of all liver symptoms is that of waking in the morning with the feeling of a mild hangover, without benefit of a previous evening's carousal. One has difficulty in waking up and wishes it were Sunday so that one could sleep an extra hour. If it is Sunday and one sleeps this extra hour it may, on occasion, make the hangover worse and even cause a mild headache.

When one gets out of bed one is stiff for the first hour.

* Taken from Arey, L. B. *Developmental Anatomy*, Figs 185 and 196A, 1946, W. B. Saunders, Philadelphia.

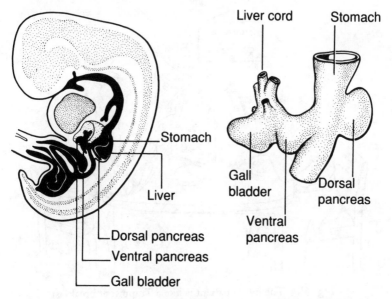

Fig. V.2

Coming down to breakfast is like walking through a mental and physical fog, and to cook a complicated breakfast would strain one's mental stamina. The ideal is to sit quietly, alone, munching one's breakfast and reading the newspaper (Fig. V.3). If one's partner comes down it is best that they do the same, for conversation jars the whole nervous system. A cup of coffee is a good stimulant, though it causes palpitations or tachycardia in some, and in the long term probably harms the liver.

Headaches and migraine

Headaches or migraine are, in my opinion, most often caused by a liver dysfunction. It is well known that an excess of alcohol, which is bad for the liver, will usually cause a hangover. Likewise, though less often, an excessively

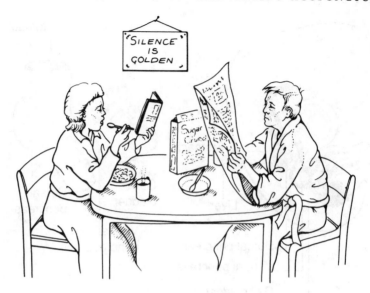

Fig. V.3 The livery patient is like a Trappist at breakfast

rich meal in the evening will in the morning cause a heavy feeling or indigestion with heartburn, which in some may be associated with a feeling of a hangover. This indigestion or hangover may progress in susceptible individuals to an actual headache or migraine.

In some people, a headache or migraine may be precipitated by lack of sleep or worry. This usually happens in patients who are primarily livery, the lack of sleep or worry acting only as a secondary stimulus. Many with headache or migraine can be cured purely by the correct dietary means, though many regard diet as a restriction of their freedom and prefer to have their liver treated by acupuncture.

The feeling of having eaten 20 dumplings

By far the most frequent digestive disturbances, in both the upper and lower abdomen, are, from my point of view, liver disturbances.

Mostly such a patient feels unduly full after a relatively small meal: the waist may actually become distended, requiring a loosening of the belt. Most typically though the patient feels full, as if he were a force-fed Strasbourg goose. Somehow this feeling of fullness extends to the whole body, so that the limbs feel heavy, the abdomen distended, breathing feels a little more laboured, the heartbeat feels more forceful and the mind seems blocked so that one has to make a greater effort to think. It is like the transformation of a light, carefree butterfly into a heavy, slightly depressed elephant (Fig. V.4). Such patients, for example, often make sure that they have only a light lunch, for otherwise they cannot work in the afternoon. If these patients have a larger, rich dinner in the evening, particularly if it is late, they may have (a) insomnia, or (b) nightmares, or may (c) stagger up to bed, feeling heavy, as if drunk, and fall into a deep, stupefied sleep, waking up the next morning, bleary-eyed, with a heavy head and slightly oedematous upper eyelids.

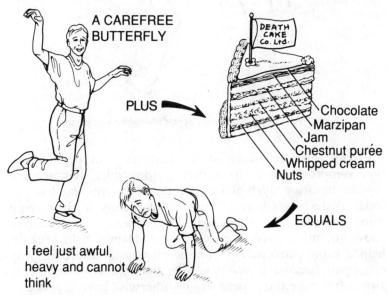

Fig. V.4 The fate of the livery food addict

Peptic ulcer-like symptoms (Fig. V.5)

Duodenal ulcers, gastritis, heartburn and related diseases or symptoms are, in orthodox medicine, often related to hyperacidity (though there is some evidence to the contrary). Hence, formerly one advocated a diet of milk, mashed potatoes and steamed fish to neutralise the acid, which only helped a minority of patients. Nowadays one may use H_2-receptor antagonists, reducing gastric acid output, which undoubtedly helps but perhaps not permanently.

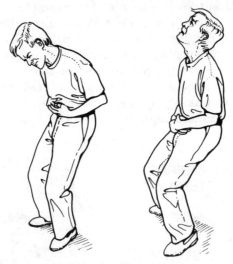

Fig. V.5 The patient with peptic ulcer-like symptoms

In my opinion, many of the patients with peptic ulcer-type symptoms are really suffering from 'liver' symptoms or 'upper digestive dysfunction'. If these patients eat less rich food, as described later in this chapter, many of their symptoms are cured or alleviated. The antacid diet mentioned above (of milk, mashed potatoes and steamed fish) probably helped some patients, not because of its acid absorbing properties but because it was less rich than the fried fish, chips and cream cake the patient might otherwise have ingested.

Eating in excess, particularly an excess of rich food, is an addiction just as difficult to break as an addiction to cigarettes, alcohol or drugs. Such patients, when under the watchful eye of their partners or in the routine of a certain job, may be able to adhere to a diet containing little rich food. However, if they go away for a weekend or to a conference or a dinner party, the temptation may prove too great and their heartburn or other symptoms start again. Taking, say, an H_2-receptor antagonist under these conditions is, I think, a good idea, though for most of the time a non-rich diet should be the mainstay of treatment which, incidentally, also reduces the incidence of other diseases.

Strange to say, acupuncture can help many liver symptoms, such as headache, migraine, dysmenorrhoea, etc., but in my experience it is of little help in most patients with peptic ulcer-type symptoms. On the other hand, H_2-receptor antagonists mostly do not help patients with headache or migraine, except for a few who have heartburn associated with a very mild headache. A non-rich diet (described later), however, can help both headache and peptic ulcer-type symptoms.

Gynaecology

Many gynaecological symptoms may be helped by treating the liver: premenstrual tension, dysmenorrhoea, menorrhagia, oligomenorrhoea, Mittelschmertz, periods which are too early or too late. However, it is best for the patient to see a gynaecologist first to ensure that no gross pathology is present.

It is interesting that treatment of the liver can help all symptoms of premenstrual tension, both the physical and mental. The swelling and tenderness of the breasts is reduced; the general feeling of, and often appearance of a swollen body are reduced; the depression, anxiety, irritability, foggy mind, inability to make decisions are all reduced or cured. Women with the severest of symptoms, who throw plates around and make hell for their beloved family, are just as easily cured as the woman with only mild symptoms (see also Chapter VI). I fondly imagine that I have saved several marriages!

The first person I ever treated by acupuncture, in 1958, was a pharmacist, whose dysmenorrhoea was so severe that she had to go to bed for 2 days a month. A single acupuncture treatment at a liver area cured her for life. This was beginner's luck, for she is a Strong Reactor (see Chapter IV). Most patients would require several treatments—and there are, of course, failures. Without this initial good result, confirming my belief in it, I would probably not have continued my studies of acupuncture.

The liver and mental symptoms

In the previous section premenstrual tension was mentioned as a condition in which the patient may have both mental and physical symptoms. Acupuncture, provided it works, can help or cure both the mental and physical symptoms in roughly equal proportions. Indeed, if one wished to treat only the physical or only the mental symptoms it would be impossible: in acupuncture one can treat both or neither.

I think there are many mental conditions which are actually nothing mental, but rather the result of a physiological dysfunction. There are, for example, some patients with hepatitis who, just before the jaundice becomes apparent, are intensely depressed, and a few are nearly suicidal. Likewise, there are some patients (but not others) who become baselessly anxious whenever they have tachycardia. This tachycardia may be caused by paroxysmal atrial fibrillation, excessive thyroxine, or even inhalation of salbutamol in a sensitive patient. The essential thing is that a physiological dysfunction has caused mental symptoms. *Ergo*, a physiological treatment may cure mental symptoms.

The reverse may also happen: a mental state causing a physical disease. The owner of a house with extensive dry rot may acquire a duodenal ulcer. Supposedly, the incidence of tonsillitis is increased in those with long-term worries.

The more usual medical teaching, that mental symptoms have mental causes, and that a physical disease is caused by physical conditions, also applies to some cases, but I suspect that the reverse applies more frequently than is supposed.

The symptoms which are most often alleviated by treatment

of the liver are *depression* and *baseless and irrational anger*. All the mental symptoms experienced in premenstrual tension may also respond. However, if someone is so depressed that they just cannot go to work, however hard they try, acupuncture is not likely to work. Some patients with depression give me the impression they are as dead as a slab of wood and that needling them is rather like driving a nail into a plank, rather than needling something alive. These patients cannot be helped, unfortunately.

Sometimes patients with anxiety or fear or phobias can also be helped when treating the liver. The most important criterion for judging this is whether or not the patient is a liver-type patient.

Other symptoms

There are numerous symptoms associated with upper digestive dysfunction or the liver (see my *Textbook of Acupuncture*, pp. 395–403). They include: dry mouth, bitter taste in the mouth, brown fur on tongue, slightly foggy vision, slight dizziness, stiff and painful neck, asthma occasionally, abdominal distension, flatus, generalised pruritus, scrotal pruritus (not pruritus ani or vulvae), rheumaticky aches and pains.

Case history. A patient had a severe scrotal itch. He worked in an open-plan office so that all and sundry could see him scratching. One of the women in the office (who was a patient) could not stand all this and sent him to me. In addition, he drank half a bottle of gin a day, and then had to stop as otherwise he would have a hangover the next day. I treated his liver on three occasions, at fortnightly intervals. Thereafter the scrotal pruritus was cured. Moreover, he could now drink not half a bottle of gin, but two bottles of gin—without a hangover.

TREATMENT OF UPPER DIGESTIVE DYSFUNCTION

Acupuncture

There are many ways of treating the 'liver' by acupuncture. My favourites are:

1 Dorsalis pedis/dorsal interosseous area.
Liv3 (LV3)
2 Lower ribs anteriorly; a large area extending say 7 cm vertically and 15 cm horizontally.
Liv14 S19 G24 (LV14 ST19 GB24)
3 Spinous processes or interspinous ligaments of T8 to T12 or the sacrospinalis at this level.
Gv9 to Gv6 and B17 to B20 (GV9 to GV6 and BL17 to BL20)
4 Sometimes a needle anywhere in the leg is sufficient; sometimes a needle anywhere in the upper abdomen, lower chest or back at the same level.

A detailed description of these acupuncture areas is given in Part II of this book. The traditional description may be read in my *Textbook of Acupuncture*.

Diet

I have many patients who are livery and, apart from acupuncture, I give them the following diet sheet (Fig. V.6).

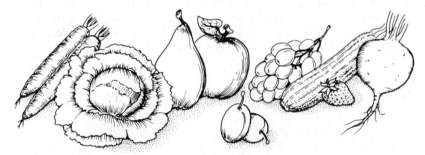

Fig. V.6 Raw fruit and vegetables is the way to heaven, but hell on earth

Rich food

Many illnesses and general ill-health in Western countries are caused, at least partially, by our Western diet, which is too 'rich'. In poor, Third World countries, with their frugal diet, some of the illnesses which we have in the West are a rarity.

Chinese medical books, written 2000 years ago, give a list of many illnesses which have a greater tendency to occur in wealthy Chinese who eat a rich diet, something a poor peasant could not do. By 'rich' was meant too much fat, oil or sweetness.

The following 'rich' items should be reduced, though not given up completely.

Fats
The fat should be cut off meat and the skin (which is fatty) should be removed from chicken. Meat consumption should be reduced a little, as there is still fat between the meat fibres. Pâté and sausages usually contain a high proportion of fat. Game, which runs or flies around in the wild, usually has less fat than farmed animals.

Milk contains a lot of fat, as may be seen from looking at a normal bottle of milk. One should therefore have skimmed milk, not semi-skimmed. Also reduce the consumption of butter, cream, cheese, yogurt made from unskimmed milk, etc.

Oils
All vegetable oils should be reduced, particularly olive oil, which is the hardest to digest. Other oils should also be reduced: corn oil, safflower oil, sunflower oil, soya oil, etc. This means a reduction of fried food, mayonnaise, French salad dressing (containing oil), margarine. Nuts and avocados also contain much oil.

Sugar
Sugar of all types (glucose, dextrose, fructose, sucrose, whether made from cane or beet, white or brown, as well as honey) should be reduced. This means no sugar in tea and coffee; also a reduction in jam, cake, biscuits, ice cream and

many soft drinks, squashes and fizzy lemonades. Remember that dried fruit contains more sugar than fresh fruit, which is why it is sweet.

Other items
All forms of alcohol, coffee and chocolate should be reduced drastically. Eggs, smoked salmon and caviar should be eaten only in moderation.

Someone who has eaten too much rich food for many years may no longer notice the effect it has on him, much as an alcoholic may drink several whiskies with little effect, whilst a teetotaller may feel the effect of a single whisky. After one has stopped or considerably reduced the consumption of rich food for several months, one may become sensitive (like a teetotaller) to rich food, so that if one suddenly consumes more than a limited amount one may feel heavy, overfull, slightly headachy, have a thick head, nausea, a dry, bitter or bad taste in the mouth, a feeling like a very mild hangover. The French would call it being 'livery'. It may occur within seconds or 24 hours of excessive consumption. This 'feeling livery' is the best guide one can have as to how much rich food one can eat or drink with relative impunity. Some people feel livery with items other than those on this list—these items should be avoided. Others never experience being livery and they cannot use this test.

Gross overeating of any type of food may have the same effect as eating moderately too much rich food.

Some people are hypersensitive to certain foodstuffs (nothing to do with rich food), chemical additives, etc. This may cause a large variety of illnesses or symptoms, and a cure depends on excluding the offending item or items. This is not the same as the intolerance of 'rich food' mentioned above, though both conditions may coexist.

I feel I am ideally qualified to write about the 'liver' as I am livery myself, and hence have repeatedly experienced many of the symptoms mentioned in this chapter. There is no need for me to read a book about the subject, for I can practically experience the symptoms within myself when patients relate their history to me.

I do not know why I am livery. I presume it might be because I grew up in an era when most people thought that rich food was good for you. Thereafter I became addicted to rich food and tended to eat more and more. If I eat a healthy meal I feel I am eating rabbit food, and if I have half a day free I feel it has not been consummated without a visit to a patisserie.

If I eat too much rich food, the following almost invariably happens, alas! I feel heavy, my brain works less well, I partially lose my mental and physical drive; I have a pain on the right/posterior side of the neck; I also have a pain on the left side of my head stretching along a line from the middle of the forehead above the eye, over the scalp to halfway along the lambdoid suture some 5 cm from the midline (corresponding roughly to part of the course of the supraorbital and greater occipital nerves or the gall bladder meridian from G14 to G19—GB14 to GB19). If this continues for a long time I have discomfort in the area of the left tonsil, as if I had mild tonsillitis; my bowel motions become slightly soft, a little pale and occasionally actually loose. I may develop acne. On occasion I may have almost any symptoms mentioned in this chapter.

This concept of the liver I find extraordinarily important in my practice of acupuncture and I am always astounded that it is hardly known in the Anglo-Saxon world. Possibly a third of my patients are 'livery' whatever else they may have in addition. It is a great pity that they remain mostly untreated due to the paucity of objective, scientific data— most doctors only believing in patients' symptoms if they can find something objective.

VI

Psycho-somatic and somato-psychic conditions

In the Western world there is a tendency to delineate sharply mental from physical disease.

Everyone knows that if one becomes bankrupt there is a possibility that one also becomes to a greater or lesser degree depressed. Most people also know that many women become depressed premenstrually, whereas during the rest of the month their mood is normal. Presumably these women's premenstrual depression is linked to premenstrual physiological changes.

It is therefore difficult to understand why so many doctors should think that practically all mental disease has a mental cause, and the reverse, that nearly all physical disease has a physical cause.

The ancient Chinese did not make this distinction. Throughout their literature one can read about the interplay of mind and body; of how, for example, cardiac function can affect the mood—and vice versa.

> 'Joy injures the heart
> Anger injures the liver
> Grief injures the lungs
> Anxiety injures the spleen
> Fear injures the kidneys.'

(From Su Wen, yinyang yingxiang dalun. Written circa 200 BC)

This goes even further for, when the ancient Chinese describe 'blood', it is difficult, if not impossible, to separate its physical function from something non-physical.

> 'The liver stores blood,
> Blood shelters the spiritual soul.'

(From the Su Wen, benshen pian)

or

> 'If Qi and blood are not evenly balanced,
> Then yin and yang will oppose one another.'

(From the Su Wen, tiaojing lun)

Formerly, similar ideas were held in Europe. One thought of four types: the melancholic or earth type, the phlegmatic or water type, the sanguinic or air type, the choleric or fire type. Each type had a characteristic physical build, temperament and tendency to certain illnesses.

As far as I am aware (Fig. VI.1):

1 A physical dysfunction can cause a physical disease.
2 A physical dysfunction can cause a mental disease.

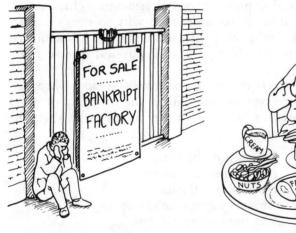
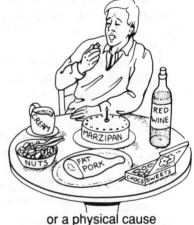

A depression may have   or a physical cause
a mental cause...   if the liver is upset

Fig. VI.1

3 A mental dysfunction can cause a mental disease.
4 A mental dysfunction can cause a physical disease.

I think that the above classification into four groups is actually rather artificial and that in reality there should only be a single group: the patient has an illness with many symptoms, some physical, some mental—the proportion varying from illness to illness and individual to individual.

Let me give some illustrations:

1 In premenstrual tension, a susceptible woman will have mental symptoms such as depression, anxiety, bad temper, crying easily, difficulty in thinking clearly, etc. She will also have physical symptoms such as retention of fluid with general swelling of the body, tender breasts, etc.

From an acupuncture point of view, premenstrual tension is a liver symptom (see Chapter V) and, if the liver is treated appropriately, the premenstrual tension is often alleviated or cured. Both the mental and the physical symptoms are alleviated or cured to roughly the same extent.

Premenstrual tension may also be helped or cured by administering the appropriate hormones or diuretics, which, like acupuncture, is a physical treatment but which helps both physical and mental symptoms.

2 Some patients with hepatitis develop a severe suicidal depression just before they become obviously jaundiced. The depression may evaporate a few days later when they actually are jaundiced.

This again is an example of a physical disease (hepatitis) causing mental symptoms (depression) and physical signs (jaundice).

3 A patient, whom I know well, occasionally has mild asthma, for which on rare occasions she needs a single puff of salbutamol. Within a very short time her asthma is alleviated, which should make her happy and relaxed. Instead she develops an uncontrollable anxiety. Examination will reveal mild tachycardia (caused by the salbutamol), which she may or may not be aware of, with possibly an associated mild discomfort in the chest.

From the point of view of traditional Chinese medicine, anxiety is linked to cardiac dysfunction. Hence in anxious

77

patients the heart should be treated, where appropriate (see Part II, Section 9).

This is an example of something physical (salbutamol) causing something else physical (tachycardia), which causes mental symptoms (anxiety)—it also helped the asthma.

4 I know someone who had dry rot in his house, which cost £80000 to eradicate. The shock was such that he had a haematemesis, causing hypovolaemic shock from which he nearly died.

In this instance a mental condition caused a physical disease and nearly death.

5 Other examples of a mental state causing a physical disease or dysfunction include: children who have a temperature before a party; people who wish to urinate or even have diarrhoea after a shock; a fright causing tachycardia, dilation of the pupil, piloerection, cold hands and feet, etc.

I think that quite a high proportion of physical disease has mental causes, and mental disease has physical causes. In my own mind I would prefer to say that much ill-health, whatever its cause, has both mental and physical symptoms in varying proportions.

In the early part of this century nearly all doctors thought that mental disease, or at least the neuroses, had a mental origin, and hence there evolved numerous schools of psychoanalysis. Nowadays the view I am expressing in this chapter is gaining ground, and pharmacists are trying to treat mental diseases with something physical: drugs.

The drugs used in this pharmacological approach have various effects on the brain. The traditional Chinese approach, however, is to treat not the physical brain but the physical organs of the body.

ACUPUNCTURE AND MENTAL CONDITIONS

Acupuncture, generally speaking, only helps the milder mental diseases, such as the mild and medium–severe neuroses, but not the severe neuroses and probably none of the psychoses.

If a patient has a neurosis so severe that he cannot go to work, or requires a supreme effort to go to work, acupuncture is unlikely to help. If the patient is psychotic and sees little green men playing football under the table, acupuncture will certainly be of no benefit.

According to Chinese tradition, dysfunction in a certain organ is liable to produce certain mental (and also physical) symptoms.

Liver and gall bladder

The most typical mental symptoms are *depression* and *irritability*. I find in clinical practice that this tradition works and it is described in detail in Chapter V.

Heart

Anxiety is the most typical symptom. What is meant by anxiety is difficult to explain but can be appreciated by any doctor who has felt anxious at the same time as he has had palpitations or tachycardia. Those who have never experienced this might like to try a little sympathomimetic. I find that treatment of the heart helps certain patients when their main mental symptom is anxiety. This is described in detail in Part II, Section 9.

Spleen and stomach

Obsession is said to be the leading symptom.

Lung

May help a few patients with *claustrophobia* or *agoraphobia*.

Kidney and bladder

Fear according to tradition is the main symptom. Children with eneuresis are possibly more frightened than other children. Many adults wish to urinate after a fright.

The above three groups, spleen, lung and kidney, I find of little use even though the link, say between the kidney and fear, may sound attractive. Hence in my actual treatment of patients I rarely use the last three groups—perhaps I do not have the appropriate skill. One exception to this is nightmares, where I find that treating the kidney is effective.

The first two groups, liver and heart, I use frequently, with good results.

Case history. A patient had for many years been mildly depressed. There was no pleasure in life—everything was grey. He wished to be by himself, particularly at breakfast. He went to work only to earn a living and at work he only did whatever he had to.

Treatment of the liver largely cured all the above symptoms. He started enjoying his work, became mentally more agile and earned more money for his firm, which in turn promoted him.

Case history. Due to the recession a patient lost his good job. He had many financial commitments, including a mortgage which had doubled due to doubling of the interest rate. He had been given a new job which involved visiting new customers to drum up new business.

He was, however, incapable of working. He was paralysed with anxiety and fear, he practically trembled the whole time, which was all painfully obvious when listening to the tone of his voice.

The heart was treated at the pisiform area on the left side only. Within a minute his facial expression changed. The next day he went out to visit new customers. His finances improved and the vicious circle was broken (Fig. VI.2).

Both of these case histories deal with patients who could not work: the former was depressed, the latter anxious. Some of their symptoms were similar, others different. Sometimes it requires considerable skill to decide to which category a patient belongs; sometimes they even belong to both simultaneously.

Both patients were a lot better after treatment, but still retained a slight tendency to depression or anxiety, as this was

A prick in the little finger
may cure anxiety.
This may enable a patient
to go back to work...

producing this for
the patient

... and this for
the doctor

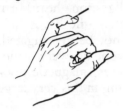

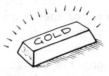

Fig. VI.2

probably their basic nature, which cannot be changed. I have the impression that many mental conditions are really a pathological exaggeration of the patient's normal temperament. A certain individual may, for example, have a very slight tendency to be depressed, but it is so slight that it does not affect his everyday life: he may indeed himself be unaware of this tendency. If such an individual is put under mental stress (or something physical affects the liver) his weakness becomes exaggerated and apparent and he becomes clinically depressed.

A psychotic, such as a manic-depressive, cannot normally be treated by acupuncture. It is interesting though that if the Chinese pulse diagnosis (see *Textbook of Acupuncture*, pp. 235–258) is performed, one finds a dysfunction of the liver in the depressive phase, which is replaced by a dysfunction of the heart during the manic phase.

PATIENTS WHO SUPPOSEDLY IMAGINE THEY ARE ILL

There are many patients who feel ill, for a longer or short period, who somewhat naturally go to see their doctor. He cannot find anything wrong—and then the difficulty arises. The patients leave with their illness the same as before, often with the additional burden of realising that their doctor thinks them neurotic. Indeed, some doctors think that more than half their patients have symptoms but no real disease.

These patients may have a large variety of symptoms: headache, fatigue—sometimes even extreme fatigue, dyspnoea, palpitations, discomfort in the chest, indigestion, heartburn, abdominal pain, diarrhoea, heavy legs, etc.—the list is infinitely long. Some of these patients may not be investigated, whilst others may be investigated with a probe up every orifice and an endless battery of blood tests, X-rays, magnetic resonance imaging, etc. The characteristic finding in this very large group of patients is precisely zero.

Since pathology became an important subject over a century ago, the thinking of doctors has changed. It is considered that one cannot have genuine disease without objective evidence of attendant pathology. This objective evidence includes histological, biochemical and chemical changes, ECG and EEG findings, etc. It is considered that there is no disease unless the physical material of the body is altered in some way—which, in practice, means a way *perceptible to doctors*.

In my opinion the above concept has two flaws:

1 Lack of knowledge

I have the impression that today we only know 10% or less of how the body functions. Every year there are new discoveries and this seems to be happening at an ever increasing rate, so that the number of medical articles published is perhaps doubled every 10 years. My mind does not stretch to what will happen in a hundred years, except that I am sure we will never know everything.

In the early part of the twentieth century, most of the tests available for diagnostic purposes were fairly crude: X-rays, biopsies and the major chemical changes in the blood, urine or faeces. These tests are quite good at detecting gross pathological changes in serious, often life-threatening diseases.

In more recent times more finely tuned and less invasive tests have been discovered: the numerous biochemical, endocrinological and immunological tests of function, magnetic resonance imaging, etc. These more finely tuned tests can often discover abnormalities which could not have been found in the early part of this century, and thus we now may have objective evidence of a disease where there was none previously. At one time epileptic patients were regarded with disdain in Europe, or as speaking the words of gods in Africa; since the discovery of electroencephalography we know epilepsy is a physical disease like any other (Fig. VI.3).

I have little doubt that, in the future, tests of a type we cannot even imagine today will be discovered. These, quite often tests of biological function, will in turn be able to demonstrate objectively a dysfunction which is not recognised today by doctors—though it is recognised by patients who feel ill. I hope that in this way patients who feel ill today, but are told they are neurotic, as all today's tests are negative, will in some instances in future be relabelled as having a 'real' objective disease.

At medical school I was taught that women with dysmenorrhoea were neurotic

Years later the 'pill' was discovered which fortuitously cured dysmenorrhoea

Suddenly doctors stopped calling their patients neurotic

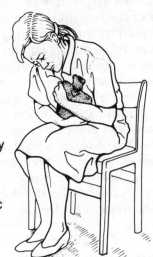

Fig. VI.3

2 *Physiological dysfunction*

It is somehow assumed by most doctors, without having thought about it too deeply, that one is either healthy or ill. I think though that there are many patients who are somewhere between these two extremes.

These in-between patients may have virtually any symptoms but, as the disease process is not advanced enough to be shown on today's laboratory tests, they unfortunately are often labelled as neurotic.

I look at the development of disease as a process in three stages:

(a) *100% healthy* This is what we should all be like, but probably few Westerners are so lucky. The unlucky ones progress to:

(b) *Physiological dysfunction* At the very early stage of a disease, whether it has a physical or mental cause, there arises a slight physiological dysfunction of the body. This dysfunction is initially so slight that it cannot be detected by today's methods of medical investigation, though, as mentioned in the previous section, the presumably more delicate tests of biological function of the future will do so.

Human beings are built in such a way that they may be extraordinarily sensitive to the slightest change in what Claude Bernard, the early physiologist, called the 'internal milieu'. I am sure that in some instances the slightest, usually undetectable, change can cause a patient to feel ill. There are many with rheumatic-type diseases who start having aches and pains a day before the weather changes; some who sleep walk or have migraine at full moon; some who feel ill with the föhn or mistral; the singers who develop a sore throat when they eat too much; those who feel revitalized after a small change in their diet.

This type of patient may feel ill for weeks, months, years or their whole life. Sometimes the dysfunction cures itself, sometimes it may progress and become a 'real' disease with an obvious physiological dysfunction, progressing to anatomical changes detectable by objective tests.

N.B. The reverse of this may also occur, for there are patients harbouring gross pathology who feel completely healthy. I remember speaking to a pathologist who, for this reason, found great difficulty in reconciling symptoms with pathology as there are also patients who are severely ill but with little to see post mortem.

The unlucky patients in this group progress to:

(c) *A real disease* The mild physiological dysfunction mentioned in (b) has become more severe, causing chemical and possibly anatomical changes in the body, which can be detected by ordinary laboratory diagnostic methods. This is now a full-blown disease which all doctors recognise.

Some diseases progress directly from (a) to (c) without going through stage (b): accidents, poisoning, etc. Acute diseases pass through stage (b) quickly: before developing flu one may feel ill for a day or two.

Acupuncture and diseases involving a mild physiological dysfunction

Acupuncture is a gentle form of treatment and hence is suitable for diseases involving a mild physiological dysfunction.

Orthodox medicine is usually more suitable for diseases with obvious irreversible pathology:

1 Surgery may remove the pathologically affected area.
2 Drugs may help as a pharmacological effect, though only rarely is there a real therapeutic cure. A patient with a peptic ulcer may take an H_2-receptor antagonist; a diabetic, insulin; the sufferer of congestive cardiac failure, digitalis. These may all help as long as they are taken every day but when treatment stops the patient's symptoms often return. Antibiotics, on the other hand, effect a real therapeutic cure.

Acupuncture can also produce a cure, but it is often in diseases where less pathology is present than in those diseases suitable for orthodox medicine. There are some doctors, of course, who would say that curing a disease which is only a mild physiological dysfunction by acupuncture is really only curing an imaginary disease by an imaginary treatment! Patients, however, think differently, as may be seen from the following case history.

Case history. A patient had typhoid fever when she was 20. I saw her first when she was 50. For the whole of these 30 years she had had virtually no energy. She worked in a museum and every day after work she went directly home, had supper and went to bed about 8.00 to 9.00 p.m. She spent more than half of her weekends in bed.

I treated her over a longer period than I do the average patient, about a dozen times. Afterwards she was, say, three-quarters cured, so that she went out in the evenings and at weekends and could enjoy life. She even said that if she had had so much energy in her twenties she would have married.

VII

Micro-acupuncture

Initially, when I started to distinguish Strong Reactors from Normal Reactors, I thought the former comprised only a small part of the population, perhaps 10%. This 10% I treated very gently.

The remaining 90%, the Normal Reactors, I stimulated more strongly, as is usual in acupuncture. At one stage I treated these patients very strongly, twisting the unpolished needled to and fro for some 2 minutes. I found later that this was unnecessary and reverted to my previous practice.

For the past few years though, I have been treating more and more patients as if they were Strong Reactors, so that now perhaps 70% of the patients in my practice are so treated.

This 70% of patients exhibit many, if not all, the characteristics of Strong Reactors:

1 Following the very first treatment there is usually some sort of response while the patient is still in my consulting room, or shortly afterwards. This response may even happen in seconds or minutes. The response may be:

(a) A feeling of relaxation, sleepiness or euphoria; occasionally laughter or crying.

(b) A temporary or permanent alleviation of whatever symptoms the patient has. The relief may encompass some or all of the symptoms.

(c) Radiation of a feeling of warmth or coolness in a distant part of the body; particularly in the affected part, if one has needled at a distant site.

2 The patients require only gentle needling at one or a few places.
3 Usually only a small number of treatments is required.

The technique of needling is similar to that for Strong Reactors.
I use a short and thin needle, usually 15 mm long and 0.2 mm
in diameter. The needle should be smoothly polished to
facilitate atraumatic needling. The point should be fine, narrow
and slightly curved, as in a sewing needle. One can use a thinner
needle but then an introducer is required, which I do not like.

If a tender area is needled, great care is needed in finding the
most tender area within perhaps a larger area which is also to
some extent tender.

The needle is inserted slowly and gently to a depth usually
of some 3 mm or less. I have the impression, but it is only a
vague impression, that, if one needles only the epidermis, the
therapeutic effect is less—the pain though may be more severe
and sharp. Needling the dermis and the most superficial part of
the subcutaneous layer seems to help more—even though the
pain of needling may be less.

The needle is removed after a few seconds.

Quite often only one place is needled, on only one side,
without using even the usual paired point. Only occasionally
are several places required.

If it is necessary to needle the periosteum, this should be
done very gently, with a gentle and slow insertion of the
thinnest needle available. The periosteum is pecked only once
or twice.

The patient should be asked to rest for a while after
treatment.

Micro-acupuncture, the name I have given to this technique, is
an enigma. Even though little is done, the results have to be
seen to be believed. Doctors who come to my acupuncture
courses are fearful that they would not be able to charge their
patients for doing so little—they think patients are impressed
by a quiverful of big, fat needles, rammed in hard and left there
for a long time, with or without the aid of grandiose electronic
apparatus. I, myself, think patients have more sense and are
perfectly capable of judging on results.

In *Scientific Aspects of Acupuncture* and elsewhere, I have described many neurophysiological experiments and measurement techniques which have a probable application to acupuncture. Whether this research is also applicable to micro-acupuncture, I do not know. It is possible that this technique might point researchers in other, even more productive, directions.

When I started practising micro-acupuncture, I did so without having given it a name, which I later realised was a great mistake. While giving a course with demonstrations in Brussels, a doctor asked what I called the technique. Without further thought I called it Casanova acupuncture, for a Casanova is more likely to be successful if he is gentle than if he is rough. My wife thought this lacking in *gravitas*: we therefore chose the name 'micro-acupuncture', as minimal dosages are its whole *raison d'être*.

There are some doctors who stimulate gently, using a needle, a laser or massage but, as far as I am aware, they normally stimulate a large number of areas. I have not heard of a technique similar to micro-acupuncture, though, admittedly, if it had no name, it might not be generally known.

Micro-acupuncture is something that just happened. I did not invent it—except in so far as it is an extension of the concept of Strong Reactors. My wife has a 'filing-system' method of recognising Strong Reactors (see Chapter IV); by combining this with my system, allied to my wife's 'nose' for Strong Reactors and also her enthusiasm, we found that an ever greater and greater proportion of patients were, or at least reacted as, Strong Reactors. From there it was but a small step to micro-acupuncture.

VIII

Periosteal acupuncture

In about 1963, after having practised acupuncture for several years, I made one of the most important inventions of my medical career—periosteal acupuncture—in which the periosteum is stimulated with an acupuncture needle.

I am not at all sure that in calling it an invention I am giving an accurate picture of what actually occurred. The process, certainly initially, was intuitive rather than cerebral. I was guided by a feeling in my hand while holding the needle, rather than by ratiocination. The nearest comparison would be to the way in which animals often appear to be guided by some sixth sense. It is my firm conviction that there are large areas of reality where logic and intellect are an important, but not sufficient, guide and that there are many ways of cognition of which the brain, the most obvious, is only one.

GENERAL CONSIDERATIONS

Nomenclature

I have called this form of acupuncture periosteal acupuncture, rather than bone acupuncture or osteopuncture, because the periosteum has a rich network of nerves, whereas the bone has a rather sparse innervation. As will be apparent from other chapters in this book, I consider the nervous system as the major substrate for the action of acupuncture and so the term periosteal acupuncture seemed the most appropriate and natural description.

A stronger effect

Some patients notice an effect with acupuncture within a few seconds of treatment (see Chapter IV). If, for example, the foot is needled, these patients will notice radiation up the leg and sometimes even up the whole body as far as the head. The further the radiation travels and the stronger and more persistent it is, the greater the curative effect.

If the periosteum is needled in these Strong Reactors, radiation is more likely to occur than with subcutaneous or intramuscular acupuncture. I have frequently needled a patient very slowly, taking, say, a minute to achieve full penetration. While the needle was in the superficial tissues, the patient would notice nothing except for the local discomfort or pain around the site of needle insertion. However, the moment that the penetration of the needle was sufficient to stimulate the periosteum, the patient noticed a result. This result might be radiation of a greater or lesser degree or, if the patient's symptoms were in, say, the neck, a reduction of pain, a greater range of movement, a feeling of warmth, or a sensation of lightness or relaxation—all in the neck or neck and shoulders.

There are, of course, some Hyper-Strong Reactors who notice all the above changes with subcutaneous or intramuscular acupuncture, but this is because these patients are so reactive that periosteal stimulation is too powerful for them and should, as a rule, be eschewed.

Normal Reactors or Hypo-Reactors may also occasionally notice the effects within seconds of acupuncture. This, however, is rare, which in turn implies that on average the treatment has a weaker effect. Note though that sometimes it is actually desirable to have a weak rather than a strong effect!

It could be thought that the enhanced effect of periosteal acupuncture is due to the increased pain which it causes. I do not think this is the case, for a subcutaneous or intramuscular needle may be twisted or pushed up and down *in situ* to cause just as much or even more pain than periosteal acupuncture, and yet the periosteal acupuncture, as a rule, will have a greater effect—I write 'as a rule' for nothing in acupuncture is absolute or 100%: it is full of exceptions and contradictions.

When I started practising periosteal acupuncture, I thought it was particularly effective in the local treatment of joints. If, for example, a patient had pain in the knee and a place nearby, say the medial infragenual area, spleen 9, was needled periosteally, the effect as a rule was greater than with more superficial needling. At that time I thought the general systemic effects with periosteal acupuncture were no greater than with normal acupuncture. I have since found that the local, distant and general effects of periosteal acupuncture are equally great.

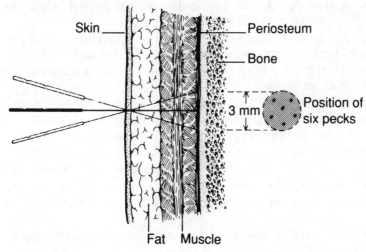

Technique of periosteal acupuncture

Technique

In periosteal acupuncture (see illustration) the needle is inserted in exactly the same way as in ordinary acupuncture. The only difference is that insertion is continued until it hits the periosteum, which, in practice, means until one hits the bone, obvious to anyone after they have done it even once.

In normal acupuncture the effect may be enhanced by twisting the needle to and fro, pushing it up and down or, for that matter, any movement.

In periosteal acupuncture, twisting of the needle has little effect on the periosteum (though inevitably it will have an effect on the skin), for the periosteum is so thin that twisting the thin tip of a needle has little extra effect. What I do instead is to peck the periosteum (i.e. the bone) like a little woodpecker. I do not peck the same place continuously but move the tip of the needle around, say, a couple of millimetres, to peck slightly different parts of the periosteum. The needle remains inserted in the same place the whole time. The looseness of the tissue in most parts of the body is such that the tip of the needle can be moved while the needle remains in the same hole in the skin.

If the patient reacts strongly to acupuncture, a single, gentle peck of the periosteum may be enough. The less responsive patient may need pecking, on rare occasions, for as long as 30 seconds.

Normally I use a thin, finely pointed, smoothly polished needle, sharpened with a curved point like a sewing needle, so that the needle slips as atraumatically as possible through the skin: thus the major part of the stimulation is periosteal though some, of course, is cutaneous and intramuscular. Mostly the needle is 0.2 mm in diameter, though sometimes it is 0.3 mm or even 0.35 mm. The length of the needle in most instances is 1.5 cm, 3 cm or 5 cm.

It is difficult or impractical to stimulate the periosteum by other means:

1 In Germany a few doctors, as far as I know, practise periosteal massage. Compressing the skin, subcutaneous tissues and muscle sufficiently to stimulate the periosteum is obviously a painful procedure and more traumatic than using a fine needle.
2 A needle can be inserted as far as the periosteum, then attached to an electrode and stimulated electrically. The electrical charge, however, would largely be dissipated in the superficial layers the needle first traverses and little electrical

charge would be left to reach the periosteum. One could, of course, use an insulated needle, as in electromyography, leaving just the tip of the needle with bare metal. This type of needle would be rather fat and painful to insert and would make a more cumbersome process out of something that is simple and takes only a few seconds.

The drawings in this book should be supplemented by constant reference to a skeleton and to anatomy atlases. A fully articulated skeleton (mine stands majestically at the top of the stairs) is particularly useful for periosteal acupuncture, as it gives a three-dimensional view, which can be surprisingly different from the flat pictures in an atlas. Moreover, it is an advantage to have more than one anatomy atlas or illustrated textbook, as the view taken and subject portrayed are often different—quite apart from individual variations in anatomy.

The radiation described and shown in drawings in the ensuing pages is merely a description of what I have noticed. The amount of variation possible is infinite, both in detail and in major ways. Indeed, the amount of variation possible is such that I was sorely tempted to describe it only in vague words with no illustrations. This elusiveness is characteristic of much of acupuncture. Hyper-Strong Reactors and even Strong Reactors can sometimes notice radiation to every single part of the body, irrespective of where they are needled, or, if they perceive radiation to only one region, that region may be in virtually any part of the body.

The tender 'areas' (not acupuncture 'points'), at which needling often has a greater effect, are likewise extremely variable in position, in size and in the shape of area covered. This variability is well known with McBurney's point or with the tenderness in the neck and shoulder in cervical disease. This variability occurs, however, with nearly all 'areas'.

If doctors notice—consistently—radiation which is different from that described in this book, I would be glad to hear of it. I would also be interested to hear both of any relatively consistent variation in position, size or shape of the tender 'areas'—and also of new 'areas'. These observations, if verified, would possibly be included in later editions of this book, suitably acknowledged.

PART II

PART II

Section 1

SACRO-ILIAC JOINT AREA
Approximately bladder 26, 27; B26, 27; BL26, 27

Low backache and sciatica may be treated reasonably success-fully by acupuncture. When I started my acupuncture practice, during the first year or two I naturally treated patients in the same way as I had been taught, which was at least partially similar to the traditional way.

The meridian of the bladder (which does not exist) runs paravertebrally over the lumbar and sacral area, where one has low backache, and then continues down the back of the thigh and calf, where one often has sciatica. The traditional theory tells one that, if there is a pain or other symptom over or near one part of a meridian, one should then needle another part of the meridian, preferably distally, such as bladder 57 in the calf (the gastrocnemius tendon area), or bladder 62 below the external malleolus (Fig. 1.1). This and other methods involving needling of distant points work reasonably well. However, one always hopes to find a better way.

I had often heard osteopaths speaking of sacro-iliac strain. Indeed, they speak about it so often that I have sometimes maliciously wondered if they know any other words in the English language. So I thought I would try the acupuncture eqivalent of osteopathic manipulation of the sacro-iliac joint by needling the area of the joint—and hey presto—I achieved better results than previously!

Needling the periosteum or bony attachments of ligaments and muscles anywhere in the lower back may help patients with lumbago or sciatica. I have tried mainly the posterior aspects of all lumbar vertebrae, the sacrum, the ileum and the ischial tuberosity (Fig. 1.2). However, some places within the square drawn in Fig. 1.2 help more than others, particularly the region of the sacro-iliac joint.

I ask the patient to sit on a chair, facing another chair (Fig.

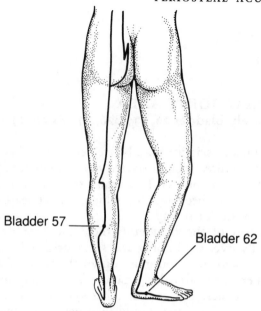

Bladder 57

Bladder 62

Fig. 1.1 Traditional treatment of low backache or sciatica

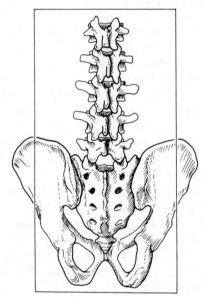

Fig. 1.2 Needling anywhere within the square may help lumbago

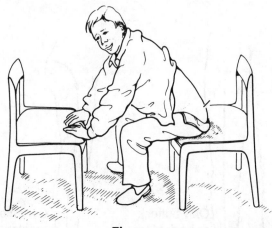

Fig. 1.3

1.3). I then ask them to lean forwards as far as they comfortably can, and rest their hands or hands and elbows on the seat of the chair in front of them. I examine the region of the sacro–iliac joint, an area about 5 cm long, which extends from the level of the spinous process of L5 to the spinous tubercles of S2 or S3. I palpate carefully the whole area of the posterior superior iliac spine, the lateral sacral crest and, between the two, the whole length of the joint, which is covered by the dorsal sacro–iliac ligament (Fig. 1.4).

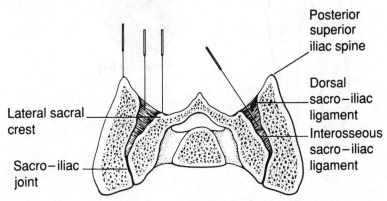

Fig. 1.4 Needling the sacro–iliac joint (transverse section)

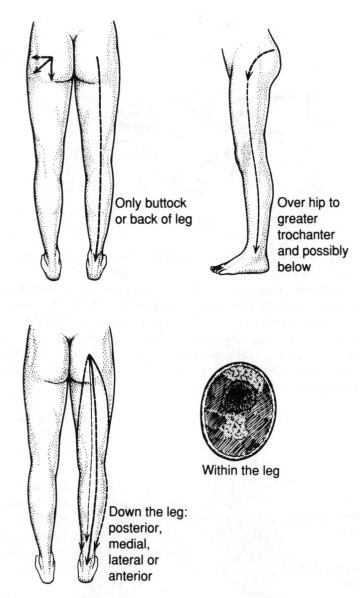

Only buttock
or back of leg

Over hip to
greater
trochanter
and possibly
below

Within the leg

Down the leg:
posterior,
medial,
lateral or
anterior

Fig. 1.5 Radiation from sacro–iliac joint

Most frequently, the posterior superior iliac spine is tender, which may be felt most easily with very light palpation, letting the fingers practically glide over the skin. Tenderness of the lateral sacral crest may be felt similarly, though less frequently. Tenderness over the joint space itself is best felt with deep, firm pressure. Tenderness is more frequently found in the upper two-thirds of the joint or surrounding bone.

I then needle the tender area, regardless of its anatomical position, until the periosteum is reached and appropriately pecked.

Sometimes, however, a tender area is not present and then either the joint or the bony prominences on either side of the joint may be needled.

Those who wish to needle the superficial fibres of the interosseous sacro-iliac ligament may place the needle at right angles to the skin. It is possible to needle the joint more deeply (which I usually do not do) by needling at 45° to the skin, pushing the needle anterolaterally, as may be seen from Fig. 1.4. I do not think, however, that the 45° needling helps more.

Radiation

The radiation which may be experienced on needling the area of the sacro-iliac joint is varied.

The commonest radiation is over the buttock, either inferiorly or inferolaterally. This radiation may extend down the back of the thigh and calf to the foot (Figs 1.5 and 1.6).

Sometimes the radiation may go down the leg medially, laterally or anteriorly. Sometimes it goes down the inside of the leg and cannot be referred to the outside. The radiation may slightly curl round the leg as it goes down.

The radiation may affect the whole foot and all the toes, though possibly the 1st toe most frequently.

The radiation may go over the hips laterally and then down over the greater trochanter, causing confusion with pain originating in the hip joint.

Rarely, there may be radiation to the lower abdomen and groin. Sometimes the pubic area, the testicles, base of the penis

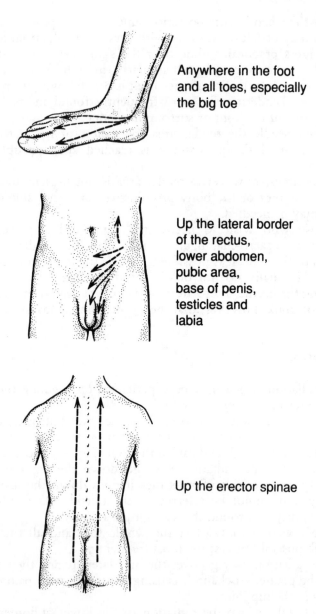

Anywhere in the foot
and all toes, especially
the big toe

Up the lateral border
of the rectus,
lower abdomen,
pubic area,
base of penis,
testicles and
labia

Up the erector spinae

Fig. 1.6 Radiation from sacro-iliac joint

or labia are affected—the most frequent cause of pain in these areas is from the back.

In a few patients, the radiation may go up the sacrospinalis to the base of the neck. Likewise, extremely rarely, the radiation may go up in the region of the lateral border of the rectus abdominis.

Frequently the radiation is not continuous but leaves out quite long sections, so that it may be felt in the buttock, to reappear below the knee, or even only in the foot.

The radiation from the region of the sacro-iliac joint is much more widespread than that from most other regions of the body, with the exception of the articular pillar of the cervical vertebrae. It may extend from the level of the navel to the ends of the toes and virtually everywhere in between.

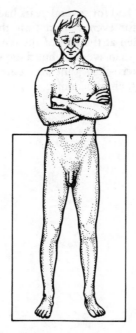

Fig. 1.7 To some extent any disease or symptom within the square may be treated via the region of the sacro-iliac joint

Diseases and symptoms which may be treated

Lower half of body

Associated with this extensive radiation, a great variety of disease within this large area (Fig. 1.7) may be treated, such as low backache, sciatica, irritable bowel, irritable bladder, prostatitis, pain in testicle or labia, gynaecological diseases, pain in knee or foot, intermittent claudication, restless legs, etc.—the list is endless. Among this long list of symptoms or diseases are some in which the treatment works well in a high proportion of cases. In others it only helps occasionally or partially, and stimulation of a different area of the body is preferable, the sacro–iliac joint area being only the second or third choice. These more practical and clinical details can only be learned satisfactorily by attending a practical type of acupuncture course.

Case history. A patient had for several years had heavy legs. Whenever she stood or walked for even a short time they became leaden and they were always leaden at the end of the day. Her hips, thighs and legs were a little fatter than average, but there was no pitting oedema.

Treatment at the sacro–iliac joint area cured the heaviness of the legs, but did not alter their appearance.

Section 2

ANTERIOR SUPERIOR ILIAC SPINE AREA
Approximately gall bladder 27; G27; GB27

Sometimes I have lumbago. I have noticed that, if I pinch the skin of the lower abdominal wall between my forefinger and thumb, the lumbago may be alleviated. Even pinching through my clothes is sufficient.

Having made this observation, I treated some patients with low backache by needling, subcutaneously, the lower abdominal wall. The needling should be below the level of the umbilicus, above the pubic hair line and medial to the anterior superior iliac spine (Fig. 2.1). This is a large area, the whole of the lower abdominal wall. It is interesting that needling anywhere in this large area has more or less the same effect, which is a further reason why I think that acupuncture points, in the classical sense, do not exist.

In this type of needling, which is subcutaneous, I use an unpolished needle that has a rough surface. If it should be

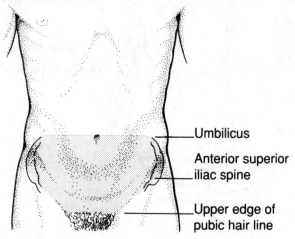

Fig. 2.1 Treatment: anywhere in shaded area

desirable to stimulate more strongly, the needle may be twisted to and fro so that the skin gripping the rough unpolished surface of the needle is twisted around with the needle.

Subsequently, I formed the impression that needling the anterior superior iliac spine has a slightly greater effect than needling the lower abdominal wall.

For this purpose, I ask the patient to lie supine and then I needle directly the most prominent part of the anterior superior iliac spine (Fig. 2.2).

Sometimes I needle from below so that the needle pierces some of the more superficial fibres of the sartorius before pecking the periosteum of the inferior aspect of the anterior superior iliac spine (Fig. 2.2).

More recently, I have found that a medial approach is the best. With the patient supine, the needle is inserted perpendicular to the skin 0.5 cm medial to the anterior superior iliac

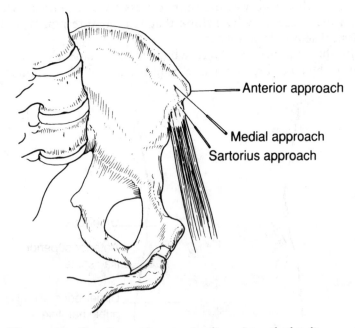

Fig. 2.2 Needling the anterior superior iliac spine and related areas

spine. The needle is then angled slightly laterally to stimulate the periosteum of the pelvic wall about 2 cm below the most prominent part of the anterior superior iliac spine. I have had several patients in whom I needled the most prominent part of the anterior superior iliac spine with little result. I then repeated the treatment a minute later, but needling medially, as described above, with a better result (Fig. 2.2).

Needling the medial side of the anterior superior iliac spine is easier in a slim patient and may be impossible in the obese. I presume that, with this technique, one stimulates branches of the iliohypogastric nerve which is L1, whereas needling at the level of the umbilicus is T10, both of which are at a higher level than might be thought appropriate—nevertheless it works.

Radiation
Diseases and symptoms which may be treated

Lower back

The radiation may be to the sacrum and lower lumbar area and hence acupuncture is of use in low backache and sciatica (Fig. 2.3).

Lower abdomen

The radiation may be to the lower abdomen, groin or, rarely, genitalia and perineum; hence needling here may be of help in symptoms in this region, such as an irritable bladder, chronic prostatitis, gynaecological disease and irritable bowel (Fig. 2.3).

Thigh

The most frequent radiation is anteriorly to the middle of the front of the thigh, which may extend as far as the knee. Needling here may help if sciatic pain, unusually, is felt on the front of the thigh. Occasionally it may help pain in the knee. It usually does not help meralgia paraesthetica (Fig. 2.3).

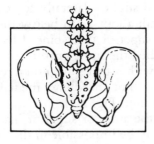

Radiation from the
anterior superior
iliac spine may go
to anywhere within
the square

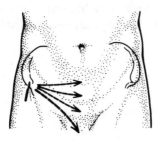

Radiation to the
lower abdomen,
pubic area,
perineum and
possibly the
genitalia

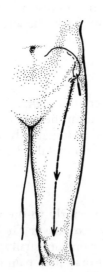

Radiation to mid–thigh
and sometimes the knee
anteriorly

Fig. 2.3

Case history. A middle-aged woman had frequent cystitis, each time successfully treated with antibiotics. Finally she was cured and her urine was sterile but she was left with an irritable bladder. She had nocturia and frequency during the day.

After needling of the anterior superior iliac spine several times she was about 75% cured.

Section 3

LUMBAR SPINOUS PROCESSES AREA
Some places correspond to standard acupuncture points

Some doctors think that the pain of low backache originates in the lumbar facet joints between the superior and inferior articular processes. W. Skyrme Rees of Australia devised a simple operation to denervate the facet joints and thus alleviate the pain. The neurosurgeon Norman Shealey introduced a modification of the above operation, involving the use of a radiofrequency probe and image intensifier. Benjamin Cox, another neurosurgeon from the USA, described to me his further modification, which required only dry needling of the facet joint.

I have further modified these three methods so that no image intensifier or other apparatus is required, for all I do is to needle the lumbar spinous processes, usually on the lateral side (Fig. 3.1).

The patient is asked to sit on a chair and lean forward, in the same way as described for needling of the sacro-iliac joint. The spinous processes can easily be palpated and then the needle is inserted 1 or 2 cm lateral to the spinous process and angled towards its base. It is easy to needle the spinous process as, in the lumbar area, it is large, a target that can hardly be missed.

The spinal cord stops at the lower border of L2. Hence, as a precaution, it is advisable when needling the upper two or three vertebrae to avoid the lamina by needling about half way along the depth of the spinous process. The lower two or three lumbar vertebrae may be needled nearer the lamina. A 3 cm needle may be used with a thin patient, whereas someone fatter will require a 5 cm needle. Sometimes I needle the tip of the spinous process or the interspinous ligament, inserting the needle through the skin in the midline. I think this helps slightly less than when needling the lateral side of the spinous process, but there is very little difference between the two methods.

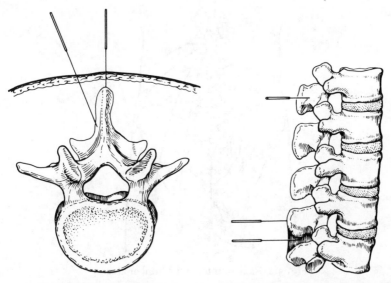

Needling the lateral side or tip of a spinous process

Lumbar spinous processes are large. Needling the lateral side, tip or interspinous ligament

Fig. 3.1 Needling the region of the lumbar spinous processes

As a rule I needle the average patient bilaterally, on the spinous processes of L3, L4 and L5.

Sometimes the sacrospinalis is tender and more prominent on one side over a length of one to five vertebrae. In that case only the tender side need be needled, intramuscularly within the tender area, though, on occasion, needling the opposite side may be more effective.

Radiation
Diseases and symptoms which may be treated

The radiation the patient perceives from needling a lumbar spinous process is usually either lateral or downwards (Fig. 3.2). It may reach as far as the iliac crest anywhere between the anterior and posterior superior iliac spines. Rarely, it may go

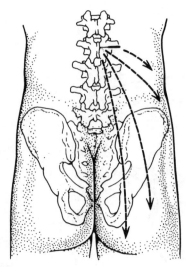

Fig. 3.2 Radiation from the lumbar area

over the whole buttock as far as the inferior gluteal fold or the region of the greater trochanter. Very rarely, the radiation goes to anywhere in the lower abdomen, genitalia or even down the legs.

It is thus apparent that the radiation can, on rare occasions, be similar to that from the sacro-iliac joint but, as a rule, there is much less and it is more localised. In my experience treatment of the sacro-iliac joint is usually the more effective option.

Case history. A patient had bilateral low backache and also pain on the right side of his neck. When the patient was standing and was examined from behind, it was apparent that his spine was leaning laterally to the left, with spasm of the left sacrospinalis in the lumbar area. There was lateral flexion of the neck on the right to compensate.

The sacrospinalis was examined and the most tender area on the left at the level of L2 was needled down to the lateral side of the spinous process of L2. After repeated treatment, both the back and neck pain were cured.

None of the methods described in Sections 1–3 help in a genuine slipped disc, spinal stenosis, or in patients who have more than a minimal neurological deficit.

Section 4

CERVICAL ARTICULAR PILLAR AREA
Does not correspond with any standard acupuncture point; Felix Mann area

In the early years of my practice of acupuncture, I used to treat patients with cervical pain, or pain of the shoulder and arm of cervical origin, by needling the dorsum of the foot at liver 3 (dorsalis pedis/dorsal interosseous area), or the front of the elbow at lung 5 (capitulum of humerus/head of radius area) (Fig. 4.1). The results were good in mild cases and in certain other instances, but failed in rather too many cases.

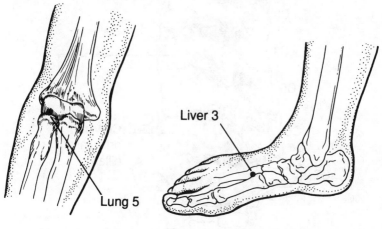

Liver 3

Lung 5

Fig. 4.1

I then discovered that needling the periosteum of the cervical articular pillar often, even if not always, produced better results (Fig. 4.2a, b).

The articular pillar is formed from the superior and inferior articular processes. It lies immediately posterior to the transverse process with its anterior and posterior tubercles. The

(a)

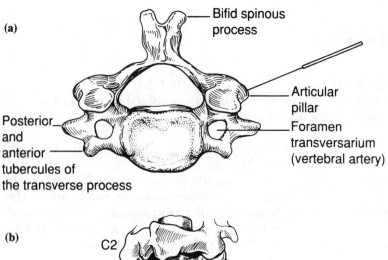

Bifid spinous process

Articular pillar

Posterior and anterior tubercules of the transverse process

Foramen transversarium (vertebral artery)

(b)

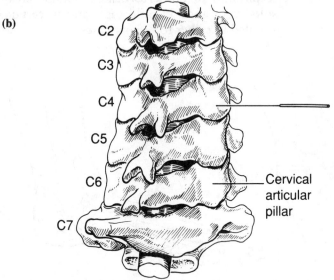

C2
C3
C4
C5
C6
C7

Cervical articular pillar

Fig. 4.2 (a) Cervical vertebra. (b) Cervical vertebrae

vertebral artery usually traverses the foramen transversarium of C1 to C6. Sometimes it may leave out the foramen of C5 and C6, in which case it lies just anterior to the transverse process. Sometimes it enters the foramen transversarium of C7. The vertebral vein consists of a plexus of veins surrounding the vertebral artery and following the same course. Due to the intricate anatomy in this area, a good atlas of anatomy and a good textbook of anatomy should be consulted before ever venturing to needle it. A skeleton, with the vertebrae in the correct position, should also be looked at.

The patient is usually sitting and I treat him standing behind him and slightly to one side (the opposite side to that which I will needle). The patient must be comfortably seated so that the cervical musculature is relaxed; this is often achieved by the patient resting his head on the doctor's chest.

The lateral side of the neck, particularly the posterolateral side, is examined, by pressing the superficial neck muscles against the articular pillar. Do not examine the anterolateral aspect as then the transverse processes rather than the articular pillar will be palpated. For some reason, at medical school, as a rule, one learns about the cervical transverse processes but not the articular pillar.

Note whichever articular pillar is tender and then needle it as described below. Most frequently the tenderness is at the level of the 4th or 5th cervical vertebra on one side. Frequently the transverse process of the atlas, which is prominent, is tender, but neither this nor the atypical articular pillar of the axis should be needled, given the proximity of the vertebral artery.

The needle is inserted over the tender articular pillar on a horizontal plane. It is then gently advanced medially and slightly anteriorly until the articular pillar is reached and pecked gently. Before insertion, the depth of the articular pillar beneath the skin should be estimated and if this is exceeded the needle should be withdrawn.

I use a needle which is 3 cm long, though less would be sufficient, and 0.3 mm or 0.25 mm in diameter. The needle should be of the finely tapered type with a polished surface, so as to needle the area as gently as possible.

Needling the neck produces fainting more often than needling other areas of the body, particularly in young men of military age. Those who give a history of fainting for any reason whatsoever, or those who are excessively nervous, should be treated lying down. In that case, the patient lies supine with the head turned to one side. I do, however, find this procedure more difficult. Since the mid-1960s I have taught this technique to several thousand doctors at my courses and lectures. I have not heard of any misadventure, other than a patient occasionally fainting.

The region of the cervical articular pillar may be stimulated more gently by needling intracutaneously, subcutaneously or intramuscularly. The cervical articular pillar may also be massaged through the overlying musculature.

Needling of the articular pillar may be used in patients who have a pain or stiffness of the neck. No obvious pathology need be present, as in patients who are tense, have been in a draught or strained their neck. It will also help even if there is a mild or moderate degree of osteoarthritis present, but is less likely to be of benefit if the patient can only turn the head 20° to the left or right. Usually the reduction of neck pain and the increased range of movement occur together, though sometimes one is helped much more than the other. The crackling sound some patients notice on turning their neck normally does not respond at once, though it may be reduced or even cease several weeks or months after the end of treatment.

Pain from the neck may often radiate down the arm (see below), in which case acupuncture may still help, though the chance of success is less than if the pain were confined to the neck or neck and shoulder.

If there are signs of a neurological deficit, acupuncture rarely helps, particularly if there are anaesthetic areas, muscle wasting or gross weakness. Paraesthesia or severe pain reduce the chance of success but not by as much as the three symptoms mentioned above. Sometimes it is very difficult to know if the pain is due to genuine nerve root pressure or is the type of pain one can have from radiation (see Chapter III), the former having a poor prognosis, the latter a much better one.

As would be expected, acupuncture does not help in spinal stenosis. It does not help in a genuine torticollis, nor for that matter in other tics, such as a facial tic, writer's cramp or a violinist's 'pearlies'.

Radiation
Diseases and symptoms which may be treated

The radiation from the articular pillar is extremely varied. It is the only place in the body, as far as I know, where radiation can occur in every direction, though more frequently in some directions than in others.

Interscapular

The commonest radiation (Fig. 4.3) is down the neck and over the back, 1 or 2 cm medial to the medial border of the scapula to the level of the inferior angle of the scapula. Often the radiation goes only as far as the superior angle of the scapula, or sometimes only reaches the base of the neck. On very rare occasions, it continues its paravertebral course to the lower thoracic or lumbar area. Frequently a 4 cm or so section is missing at the top of the shoulder.

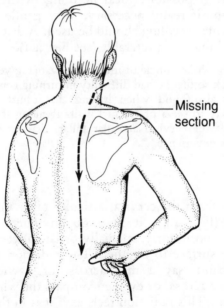

Missing section

Fig. 4.3 Radiation down the back

Given the approximate area traversed by or near to the radiation, the following symptoms or diseases may be treated: pain in the lower part of the neck with pain or limited movement laterally or posteriorly; pain over the shoulder or interscapular area. However, only on very rare occasions is paravertebral pain in the lower thoracic or lumbar area helped.

I find that interscapular pain responds more often to cervical treatment than to local interscapular treatment of the muscles or upper thoracic vertebrae. I believe that osteopathic doctors find the same.

Whiplash injuries may respond to the same treatment, particularly if they are mild. The more severely affected patient who, much of the time, has dizziness, headache, pain in the back and front of the neck, shoulders, etc. responds less well. I presume this is possibly due to the irreversible pathology which includes microhaemorrhages and micronecrosis throughout the neck, the soft tissues, the bone and even the spinal cord. Quite often the neck is excessively tender in this type of patient. Therefore, if possible, local needling of the neck should be avoided, or if really necessary, very gentle subcutaneous or intramuscular needling should be used. A distant point, such as liver 3 or lung 5, is preferable (see Fig. 4.1).

Case history. A late uncle of mine, of advancing years, had a stiff and painful neck so that he had difficulty in turning round when reversing his car. He also found, when driving, that it hurt when he turned his neck quickly to see a pretty girl walking along the pavement. After needling of the cervical articular pillar, driving became more of a pleasurable experience.

Arm

Radiation from the cervical articular pillar may also go down the arm (Fig. 4.4). It may go anywhere down the arm: anteriorly, posteriorly, medially or laterally, or alter its course from one surface to another. The radiation may consist of a narrow band, say 2 mm across, or a wider band several centimetres across, or even encompass the whole of the surface of the arm. This radiation feels as if it is in the surface or near the surface (Fig. 4.5a). The radiation may also feel as if it is

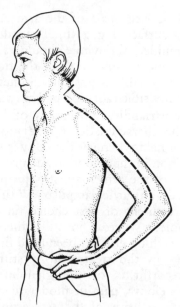

Fig. 4.4 Radiation may go anywhere in the arm

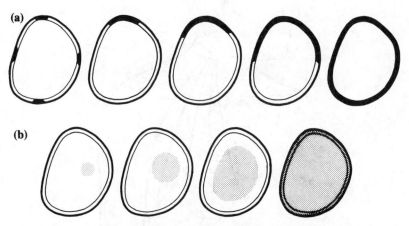

Fig. 4.5 (a) Radiation may be a narrow, wide or a complete band on the surface (transverse section of arm). (b) Radiation may be internal, along a narrow 'channel', a wide 'channel', or occupy the whole arm

inside a small or large part of the arm and cannot really be localised on the surface (Fig. 4.5b). The radiation may go across part of the shoulder, the whole shoulders, to the upper arm, the lower arm and to any or all of the fingers. Nearly every combination imaginable is possible. Sometimes small or large sections of the invisible radiation pathway are missing.

This infinite variability and variety of radiation is a general principle of the characteristics of radiation, being applicable within a certain field wherever the body is needled.

As the radiation in the arm is so all encompassing, it follows that *all* disease of the arm may, if appropriate, be treated by needling the cervical articular pillar. With some conditions it may be the treatment of first choice, in others it may be a reasonable choice, whereas in still others it is only worth needling if everything else has been tried first.

It may help in the treatment of stiff shoulders, frozen shoulder, osteoarthritis of the glenohumeral joint, tennis elbow, golfer's elbow, pain or moderate swelling in the wrist or fingers, osteoarthritis of the 1st carpometacarpal joint. It

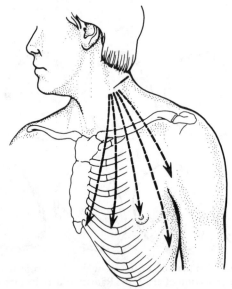

Fig. 4.6 Radiation in the chest

may help in Raynaud's phenomenon or generalised swelling of the fingers of unknown cause.

Unusual patients with a, presumably, mixed neurological and vascular pathology may also be helped.

Case history. A patient had pain and tingling in his right neck, arm and hand. When he straightened his neck and thoracic spine the tingling in the right hand became worse, with swelling of the superficial veins of the hand. This was all about 90% cured by needling the neck.

Doctors who practise acupuncture often see patients who do not fit the specific pigeon-holes into which they are 'supposed' to fit and who then unfortunately may be labelled neurotic; a label which follows them from doctor to doctor, who write polite coded letters to one another. Some of these patients may be helped by acupuncture and, if the symptoms or pathology are in the arm, treatment of the neck may provide the answer.

Chest

Radiation from the cervical articular pillar may also go to the chest anteriorly (Fig. 4.6). The radiation may go from the midline over the manubrium, sternum and xiphoid process to the lateral chest wall. It may reach from the area of the clavicle above to the level of the male nipple below. Medially the radiation may reach the xiphisternal joint. Laterally the radiation may extend further, from the axilla to the tip of the 12th rib. As is usual, the radiation may follow narrow lines—as in the mythical meridians—but often not following the classical course. At other times there may be a broad sheet of radiation covering a quarter, half or all the chest wall. Sometimes the radiation feels as if it is inside the chest and cannot be localised on the surface.

I have had several patients with cardiac-like symptoms in the upper half of the chest, which may or may not be brought on by exercise or emotion. Naturally they have seen a cardiologist, who found the ECG and other tests normal. By exclusion, and with great regret, the patient is then labelled more or less as neurotic. Patients of spirited or fiery temperament promptly label the cardiologist an 'insolent know-all' and just as promptly visit someone who practises unorthodox medicine. On the other hand, if the patient is meek or overawed by the medical profession's knowledge, he might sink into utter dejection. This is the sad background of some of the 'cardiac' patients I see. I personally prefer to tell a patient that I do not know this or that, rather than putting the blame on to the patient and labelling him neurotic. Needling the neck, usually accompanied by a few words of reassurance, cures some of these patients.

A cardiologist may say that I have merely 'cured' a neurosis —no mean feat in itself in my view—and not a cardiac disease. I tend to think that the patient had a mild physiological dysfunction of the heart which caused symptoms but did not affect the various laboratory techniques known to cardiology.

I remember another patient who frequently had paroxysmal auricular tachycardia, necessitating several short stays in hospital. He also had a stiff and painful neck. Needling the cervical articular pillar cured him of both conditions.

Tietze's disease may affect the osteochondral junction of some or all ribs. Needling the neck may help or cure this condition—though it must be said that sometimes there are other or better ways of treating it.

The pain of postherpetic neuralgia, if it occurs on the chest and has not been present for more than a few weeks or months, may likewise be partially or totally alleviated.

Sometimes the pain of chronic pancreatitis may be felt in the lower chest anteriorly or laterally and this may respond, at least partially, to neck treatment. There are, however, other more effective ways of treating it by acupuncture.

There are many vague and not so vague pains and aches patients may have in the chest. Sometimes these are called intercostal neuralgia, Bornholm's disease, muscular rheumatism, etc. These may also sometimes respond to neck treatment.

Neck and head

Radiation from needling the cervical articular pillar may also go upwards. However, this is less frequent than the downward radiation, down the arm, the back or the chest wall, mentioned previously.

The most frequent radiation in an upward direction is up the posterolateral side of the neck and over the occipital and parietal area (Fig. 4.7). Usually the course is over the superior temporal line or possibly 1 or 2 cm above (the temporalis muscle is attached to the inferior temporal line and the temporalis fascia to the superior temporal line). Less frequently, or rarely, the radiation may go to virtually anywhere in the neck and head, almost always on the same side as the needling.

A less frequent or even rare radiation may be to the area of the sternoclavicular joint, the front of the neck generally, the larynx or the base of the tongue (Fig. 4.8).

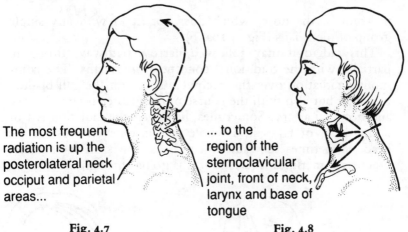

The most frequent radiation is up the posterolateral neck occiput and parietal areas...

... to the region of the sternoclavicular joint, front of neck, larynx and base of tongue

Fig. 4.7   Fig. 4.8

Sometimes the radiation may be to the front of the ear and temple or even to the maxilla (Fig. 4.9).

The most frequent upward radiation, as mentioned above, is up the posterolateral aspects of the neck, the occiput and parietal area, corresponding more or less, for those who believe in them, to the course of one or other of the gall bladder meridians. Rarely, this radiation may continue forwards to the region of the frontal eminence, the frontal sinus, the eye and

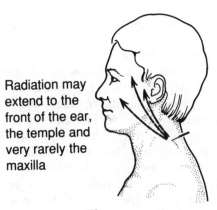

Radiation may extend to the front of the ear, the temple and very rarely the maxilla

Fig. 4.9

the root of the nose, which does not fit in with any single group of meridians (Fig. 4.10a, b).

This radiation may follow a narrow pathway, fitting in partially with the traditional concept of meridians. The commonest radiation over the occiput fits in with the gall bladder meridian but also with the course of the greater occipital nerve and occipital artery. Sometimes, however, the radiation is 1 or 2 cm wide, or takes in a whole section or even most of the head. Sometimes the radiation feels as if it is on the surface, whereas sometimes it feels as if it is going through the head or

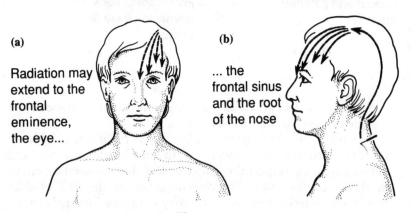

(a)

Radiation may extend to the frontal eminence, the eye...

(b)

... the frontal sinus and the root of the nose

Fig. 4.10

brains. The radiation may be continuous or it may leap-frog over small or large sections.

The diseases or symptoms in the head and neck which may be treated following this widely variable pattern are equally variable. To some extent all diseases or symptoms of the head and neck may be treated (which reminds me of the time when tranquillisers were given to all and sundry), though in some it has little effect or only rarely a good effect.

The commonest condition treated, following these radiation patterns, is pain or discomfort at the back of the neck and occiput. This may be expanded to include most varieties of headache and migraine. Care should be exercised in diagnosis, however, as the symptoms of secondaries in the brain may be alleviated for 3 days. Cluster headaches respond only occasionally unless they are relatively mild. The unfortunate patients who have a headache 24 hours a day, 365 days a year for several years, likewise rarely respond: they may have a food intolerance and should be treated with the appropriate diet (see Chapter V).

Pain over the frontal sinuses, whether or not there be an infection, may respond. Pain in and around the eye may likewise respond, though again care should be taken in diagnosis as most doctors, including myself, know little about genuine ophthalmological diseases.

Symptoms in front of the ear, of the temporomandibular joint, pain in the temple (but not temporal arteritis), pain over the maxilla, nasal symptoms and occasionally even non-specific toothache may all respond.

Symptoms over the front of the neck may likewise respond: a feeling of constriction in the throat; singers whose voices give out after singing only a short while or who have difficulties with the upper or lower register. However, aphonia rarely responds.

Dizziness as well as mild vertigo without nystagmus may be alleviated. The vertigo and nausea component of Ménière's syndrome may be likewise alleviated, though the tinnitus and deafness remain the same.

It is thus apparent that needling the cervical articular pillar may, if appropriate, have an influence which is greater, in my

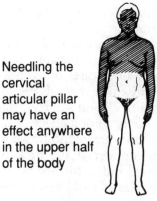

Needling the
cervical
articular pillar
may have an
effect anywhere
in the upper half
of the body

Fig. 4.11

experience, than that of nearly all other so-called acupuncture points. It may indeed be used to treat any disease or symptom in the upper half of the body above the diaphragm: the head, neck, chest and arms (Fig. 4.11). An Egyptian orthopaedic surgeon who, apart from his orthopaedics, practises acupuncture, told me that he could make a good living using no acupuncture points whatsoever apart from this one. He called it the Felix Mann point. I am indeed proud to have discovered the periosteal needling of the cervical articular pillar, which I have not seen described anywhere else in the Chinese or Western literature.

Why is the field of influence so large with this (non-existent) acupuncture point or area? I do not know. Possibly it is related to the unusually large concentration of sympathetic ganglia and sympathetic nerve fibres in the area. There are the superior cervical ganglion (C1 to C4), the middle cervical ganglion (C5 to C6) and the stellate or cervicothoracic ganglion (C7, C8, T1)—all with variations. There are numerous sympathetic fibres connecting the ganglia and coursing throughout the whole region. I think that these cervical sympathetic fibres, whose further course is often perivascular, innervate most structures in the upper half of the body. According to my theory, the acupuncture needle stimulates the sympathetic afferent fibres (not the more familiar efferents) and it is this stimulation that causes the radiation often felt on needling (see Chapter III).

As a rule, if a patient has symptoms on the right side of the neck or head, or in the right arm or chest, palpation reveals tenderness of the articular column also on the right. Sometimes, however, the tenderness of the neck is on the opposite side to the side of the symptoms. If the tenderness and symptoms are on the same side, I of course needle the tender side. if they are on opposite sides, I usually needle the side of the neck which is tender. However, there are no hard and fast rules in acupuncture and, in this case also, occasionally doing the very opposite helps more.

Section 5

DORSALIS PEDIS/DORSAL INTEROSSEOUS AREA
Liver 3; Liv 3; LV3

Liver 3 is one of my favourite (non-existent) acupuncture points or areas. In fact there are several doctors who say I know nothing about acupuncture apart from liver 3. I use it every day as it has such a universal application, which may be appreciated by reading Chapter V.

The position (Fig. 5.1) which I normally use is on the dorsum of the foot between the 1st and 2nd metatarsals, where the dorsalis pedis artery and vein turn into the sole of the foot between the two heads of the 1st dorsal interosseous muscle.

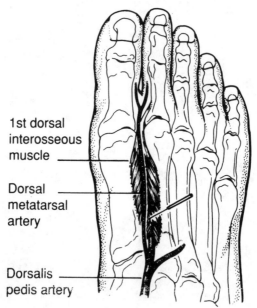

Fig. 5.1 Dorsalis pedis/dorsal interosseous area or liver 3

Medially is the tendon of the extensor hallucis longus, laterally the 1st tendon of the extensor digitorum longus. The tendon of the extensor hallucis brevis may cross the area. The medial terminal branch of the deep peroneal nerve may be medial or lateral. In the sole of the foot the dorsalis pedis artery meets the deep plantar arch. Some authors position the point also between the 1st and 2nd metatarsals but 1 or 2 cm further distal.

The needle pierces the skin in this position and is then inclined medially to hit the periosteum on the lateral side of the 1st metatarsal.

At one time, instead of needling liver 3 I needled the end of the big toe in some 20 consecutive patients (Fig. 5.2). This position is not an acupuncture point, yet the result, as far as I could tell, was the same as that achieved when needling the dorsalis pedis/dorsal interosseous area. It is of course possible that there was a slight difference I did not detect but, if so, it was so slight as to be of little clinical importance. Possibly needling anywhere in the medial and distal half of the foot would have the same effect; possibly needling anywhere over a much larger area would likewise have more or less the same effect. There are endless contradictions (see Chapter II).

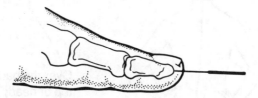

Fig. 5.2 Experimental alternative to liver 3

Radiation

The radiation that may be experienced varies. It may occur for only, say, a centimetre around the needle. It may go into the big toe or, extremely rarely, into the 2nd toe. It may go up the medial side of the foot. It may go to the sole, staying on the medial side or going across to the lateral side (Fig. 5.3).

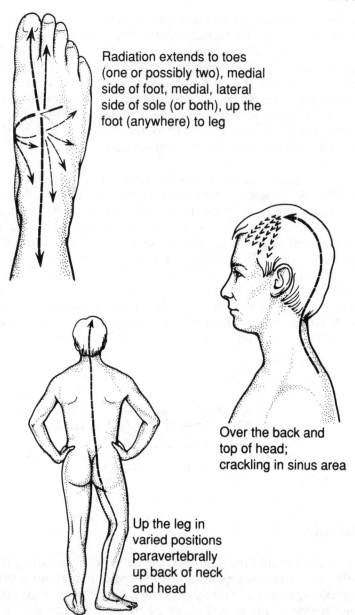

Radiation extends to toes (one or possibly two), medial side of foot, medial, lateral side of sole (or both), up the foot (anywhere) to leg

Over the back and top of head; crackling in sinus area

Up the leg in varied positions paravertebrally up back of neck and head

Fig. 5.3 Radiation from dorsalis pedis/dorsal interosseus area

The more distant radiation goes up the leg. The liver meridian, according to traditional books, runs up the medial side of the lower leg and thigh to the groin. The radiation, however, as a rule 'just runs up the leg' in such a way that many patients have difficulty in localising it more precisely. It runs just as often inside the leg, in which case it cannot be correlated with any surface markings. If it runs near the surface, it may do so medially, laterally, anteriorly or posteriorly; perhaps slightly more frequently, medially and anteriorly and least often posteriorly. The radiation, whether on the surface or in the interior, may be a couple of millimetres across or occupy a quarter, half or all the leg (Fig. 5.3).

In the stronger reactors the radiation may continue up the body, in which case it usually runs up the sacrospinalis, though it is not unknown for it to run ventrally, usually in an indefinite way. Thereafter, as a rule, it runs up the back of the neck, over the occiput to the top of the head, after which it can produce a crackling sensation in the middle of the head, presumably related to the sinuses. At the same time, the neck and shoulders may feel relaxed, the cheeks become pink and the eyes feel unusually clear.

It is thus apparent that the radiation up the leg occasionally corresponds to the course of the main liver meridian, but usually it does not or does so only partially. Radiation continuing up the trunk, neck and head does not really correspond at all, except occasionally, with the course of the main liver meridian nor, for that matter, with the branches of the main liver meridian, the liver divergent meridian, connecting meridian or muscle meridian (see *Textbook of Acupuncture*, pp. 394, 402–403, 454–457). Nor does it correspond with the course of the allied gall bladder meridian series.

Diseases and symptoms which may be treated

The diseases and symptoms that may be treated by stimulating the area of liver 3 are almost all-embracing. It is one of the few places in the body which if stimulated, even unilaterally, can produce, in a Strong Reactor, a sensation in the whole body on

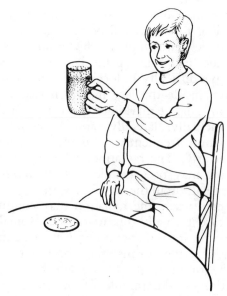

Fig. 5.4 Beer, or for me, liver 3 'refreshes all the parts'

both sides. This all-enveloping sensation can, of course, occur by needling quite a number of other places, but with the dorsalis pedis/dorsal interosseous area it is by no means a rare phenomenon. It is for this reason that symptoms in all regions of the body may be treated by liver 3. In some instances liver 3 is the treatment of first choice, whereas in others, where it has a slighter effect, it is only worth trying if other methods have failed. Like the beer, 'it refreshes all the parts'; indeed, if a patient feels just 'run down', the cause as likely as not, in a Westerner, is a mild liver dysfunction, and needling liver 3 may answer very well (Fig. 5.4).

Like the French, I ascribe a whole multitude of diseases and symptoms to the liver and have, therefore, devoted a separate chapter (Chapter V) to it. The symptoms that may be treated via liver 3 are described further in that chapter.

Section 6

MEDIAL INFRAGENUAL AREA
Approximately spleen 9; Sp 9; SP9

Some painful conditions of the knee respond to needling the medial infragenual area (Fig. 6.1).

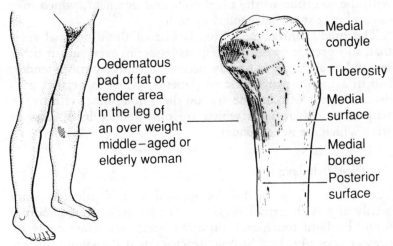

Fig. 6.1 Upper part of medial aspect of the tibia showing the infragenual area

This area is below the knee, medially. It is *visible* in middle-aged or elderly women who are overweight. These women have a slight oedematous swelling in the area shown, an area the size of a large hen's egg. When palpated, the whole or only a small part of the egg-sized area may be tender. Sometimes several small areas within the total area are tender, the remaining parts being normal or near normal. Men, younger women or slim women have exactly the same areas of tenderness but usually do not have the oedematous swelling.

Within this large area, the place most frequently tender is the

135

osseous medial border of the tibia. Anterior to the medial border lies the medial surface, which is the second most commonly tender area—again osseous. Posterior to the medial border is an area which is soft on palpation, consisting of the sartorius, gracilis, semimembranosus, semitendinosus and medial head of the gastrocnemius. This soft, posterior area may also contain a tender area, but less frequently than the osseous areas mentioned above, i.e. the medial border or the medial surface.

Formerly I thought this egg-shaped tender area corresponded with the insertion of the tibial collateral ligament, which may have a bursa superficial and deep to it.

The medial infragenual area is one of these unusual areas that, to a greater or lesser extent, is tender in everyone of either sex and at any age. It merely becomes relatively more tender, and in a higher proportion of patients, when associated with disease. Areas of this type are, on the whole, more effective in acupuncture than areas which are only tender in disease, or areas which are never tender.

Treatment technique

The whole of the medial infragenual area is palpated, both gently and with firmer pressure. Tender areas are sometimes found by light touch and, on other occasions, more easily by heavier pressure. In a Strong Reactor, or if the symptoms are very mild, merely intracutaneous or subcutaneous needling, with a thin needle, may be sufficient. In most other cases, periosteal needling of the most tender area is required. Most frequently, this is the medial border of the tibia, particularly where it is curved, just below the condyle of the tibia. The second most frequently tender area is the medial surface of the tibia. The least frequently tender area is in the muscles posterior to the medial border. In this last instance, the needle should be inclined anterolaterally, so that after the soft tissues have been pierced, the periosteum of the posterior surface of the tibia is stimulated.

There is a Chinese acupuncture point called spleen 9 within the medial infragenual area. In the vast majority of Chinese books, it lies in the soft area posterior to the medial border of the tibia, as may be seen in their illustrations and also inferred from the fact that they usually say it should be needled to a depth of one to three Chinese inches, which is clearly impossible when needling the medial border or the medial surface. Possibly the Chinese preference for the intramuscular area is due to their horror of periosteal acupuncture: they throw up their hands in shocked disapproval whenever my colleagues go to China and mention it.

Radiation
Diseases and symptoms which may be treated

The radiation from the medial infragenual area is perhaps less marked than that from some other areas (Fig. 6.2).

It may radiate down the medial side of the leg to the ankle and foot. It may thus be used to treat painful conditions of the ankle or foot, particularly on the medial side. This could

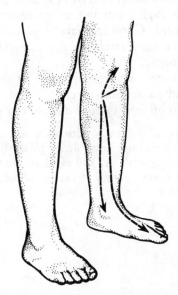

Fig. 6.2 Radiation into ankle and foot and into the knee joint

include a sprained ankle with pain on the medial side, mild pain from a bunion or pain from a dropped longitudinal arch.

The radiation may also go right into the knee joint itself. Sometimes it feels as if it is on the surface and sometimes as if it is right inside the knee. The medial infragenual area is by far the most important area for treating the knee itself. In this respect, at least in my experience, it is more effective than all other acupuncture points or areas added together. As far as the knee is concerned, it is of benefit not only if pain is on the medial side of the knee, but also nearly as effective if the pain is on the lateral side, or, for that matter, anterior or posterior.

Clearly acupuncture cannot help if there are too many gross pathological changes. Thus it may help in mild osteoarthritis or the rarer condition of a mild burnt-out rheumatoid arthritis. I suspect it might help in a mildly torn medial or lateral cartilage, but certainly not in a severe one. Often the patient has a mild pain in the knee, especially when straining it, and the rheumatologist or orthopaedic surgeon is at a loss to find a cause: this type of problem is more likely to respond to acupuncture. If there is reduced flexion at the knee joint, it may respond if it is slight, but not when severe. A hydroarthrosis does not respond. Chondromalacia patellae does not respond or does so only very rarely in my experience, though others are more optimistic.

In short—in my experience, some of the milder knee conditions respond to acupuncture. It is not, however, an area I would treat too often if I could choose my patients freely.

Case history. One of my early patients was a clergyman who, for a year previously, could not kneel down to say his prayers. Treatment at the medial infragenual area did not cure him, but at least enabled him to bend his knees enough to say his prayers while kneeling on a 15 cm high cushion.

Section 7

GASTROCNEMIUS TENDON AREA
Including bladder 57, 56; B57, 56; BL57, 56

The gastrocnemius tendon area (Fig. 7.1) is a large area
extending from the middle of the gastrocnemius muscle to
the middle of the calcanean tendon, a distance of 15 cm or a
little more. The upper part lies in the midline posteriorly, in
the region of the tendinous raphé between the heads of the

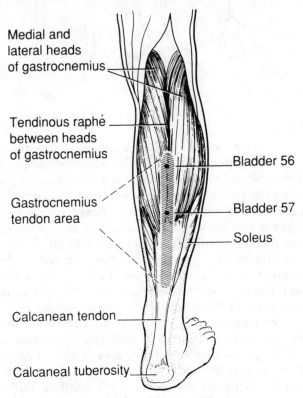

Medial and lateral heads of gastrocnemius

Tendinous raphé between heads of gastrocnemius

Gastrocnemius tendon area

Bladder 56

Bladder 57

Soleus

Calcanean tendon

Calcaneal tuberosity

Fig. 7.1 Gastrocnemius tendon area

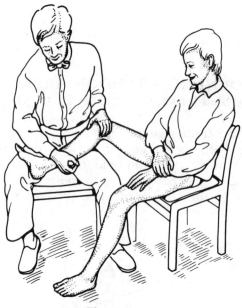

Fig. 7.2

gastrocnemius. It extends down, again in the midline posteriorly, into the tendo calcaneus. The width of the tender area
in both muscle and tendon varies, though it is usually 3 cm.

Examine the patient's leg in the position shown in Fig. 7.2,
with the knee and the ankle slightly flexed to produce some
tension in the calf muscles. The doctor should sit comfortably
in a chair with the patient's leg across his thigh. If the correct
degree of pressure is applied to the foot, several tender areas
become apparent in the area shown. These areas are no longer
apparent if the pressure on the foot is too great or too little.

In some patients the whole of the gastrocnemius tendon area
is tender, an area about 15 cm long and 3 cm wide. In others
only one or two small areas within this large area may be
tender. The gastrocnemius tendon area is one of those, relatively few, areas which is tender in all people in both health
and disease. As mentioned previously, needling this type of
area is particularly effective. Needling may be subcutaneous,

intramuscular or even deeper, to stimulate the periosteum of the posterior surface of the tibia. In most parts of the body needling the periosteum has a greater effect than needling more superficial areas but, for unknown reasons, this is not the case with the gastrocnemius tendon area.

Radiation

Radiation (Fig. 7.3) may be down the back of the calf, into the ankle and foot. It may go up into the knee and thigh. Radiation from the gastrocnemius tendon area is less marked than from many other areas and, when it is present, is rather vague, so that the patient has difficulty in describing its position and extent.

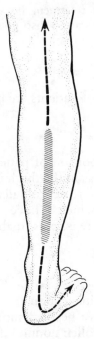

Fig. 7.3 radiation to back of calf, ankle, foot; also into knee and thigh

Diseases and symptoms which may be treated

Intermittent claudication

Acupuncture works very well in some patients and is a failure in others. I imagine it is effective in those patients in whom a major component of their symptoms is vascular spasm and is a failure in those in whom the major component is organic narrowing.

The narrowing of the arteries in intermittent claudication is usually at a higher level than that at which the pain is located in the calf; indeed it is often in the external iliac artery. At one time, therefore, I tried needling equivalent positions at the back of the thigh or buttocks or lower back. The results were no better, perhaps even a little worse, and so I have gone back to needling the gastrocnemius tendon area.

Case history. A patient had to stop walking after 50–100 metres. Immediately after the first treatment he walked home—some 10 kilometres! Normally results are not so good or dramatic, but they are the ones I remember!

Night cramps

A reasonable proportion of patients are helped.

Restless legs

Again, a reasonable proportion of patients are helped. Sometimes needling tender areas in the thigh in addition will help. It does not help in the very rare neurological disease called restless feet and moving toes, which I have tried to treat in three patients, but in which there is, presumably, irreversible pathology present.

Achilles tendonitis

Needling the gastrocnemius tendon area may help dramatically in some patients. The area needled should be 10 cm or more away from the tender swollen nodule. If the nodule itself were needled it might cause a flare-up.

In addition to needling the gastrocnemius tendon area, one may needle anywhere at the back of the heel to stimulate the periosteum on the posterior surface of the calcaneus.

Case history. I had a patient with bilateral Achilles tendonitis who could only go upstairs, backwards on all fours. Three treatments at only the gastrocnemius tendon area cured him.

Plantar fasciitis

Needling the gastrocnemius tendon area may help or cure patients with plantar fasciitis. It may even help in some patients where a local steroid injection has failed.

Sometimes I needle the tender area directly (see Section 14). This is usually situated in the region of the anterior tubercle on the plantar surface of the calcaneus. Alternatively, the medial and lateral processes of the calcaneal tuberosity may be needled from the medial or lateral side (see Section 14).

Circulatory changes

Some patients, particularly women, may have bluish feet. Needling the gastrocnemius tendon area may help in a small or perhaps very small proportion of patients. It is not worth asking patients to come for treatment if they only have this condition. It is only worth trying if the patient has a concurrent disease in which the chance of success is fairly high.

Generalities

Needling the gastrocnemius tendon area may help various symptoms which, however vague, may cause great discomfort to the patient, such as a heavy feeling in the calf or feet or legs in general, as if they were made of lead; or odd aches and pains in the calf or feet. All these symptoms may also be helped by needling the sacro-iliac joint area.

It is thus apparent that the gastrocnemius tendon area has a fairly wide application. Many of the areas for needling described in this book have a broad field of action, and therefore, generally speaking, they are of more use therapeutically.

Section 8

VARICOSE ULCER AREA
Corresponding roughly with spleen 6, 7, 8; liver 5, 6; kidney 8
Sp6, 7, 8; Liv5, 6; K8; SP6, 7, 8; LR5, 6; K18

This is a large tender area, tender in most people, of either sex, in both health and disease. The area is extremely variable in size and shape, ranging from a spot the size of a pea to a major portion of the leg (Fig. 8.1).

Perhaps the most characteristic place in this area corresponds roughly to the well-known classical Chinese point called spleen 6. This fits in, more or less, with the amazingly constant position of a varicose ulcer, which occurs where a perforating

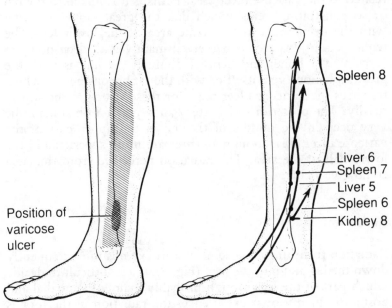

Fig. 8.1 Varicose ulcer area

vein connects the great saphenous vein with the posterior tibial veins. It is for this reason that I call this whole area the varicose ulcer area.

The varicose ulcer area is bounded above by a line some 5 cm below the lower border of the tibial tuberosity, whereas below it is bounded by a line some 2 cm above the most prominent part of the medial malleolus. The whole area is about 4 cm wide. In the upper part of its course, 3 cm of this is posterior to the medial border of the tibia, whereas anteriorly it extends from the medial border of the tibia about 1 cm across the medial surface of the tibia. In the lower part of its course the area posterior to the medial border of the tibia becomes only 1 cm wide, whereas anteriorly it covers most of the medial surface of the tibia.

As mentioned above, the whole of the varicose ulcer area is tender in most people, of either sex. This tenderness is, however, particularly marked in women.

It is difficult to name any particular anatomical structure related to the varicose ulcer area. Perhaps it is linked to the ten or so penetrating veins which link the great saphenous vein with the deep veins in this same area of the lower leg. The tenderness in this area is perceived mainly with deep pressure (except over bone) and hence I doubt if the link is with the great saphenous vein itself or with the saphenous nerve, which traverses the varicose ulcer area, for these structures lie superficially. The posterior tibial artery and vein and tibial nerve lie very deep in the middle of the leg in the upper part of the varicose ulcer area, though all three are more superficial in the lower half of the area. The radiation perceived from this area could give a clue.

Radiation

Radiation from the varicose ulcer area extends most frequently down the leg and into the foot (Fig. 8.2); it is difficult to decide which part of the leg, though probably mainly the medial and posterior. In my own experience, the radiation in the foot is along the whole sole, though others notice it in the toes only.

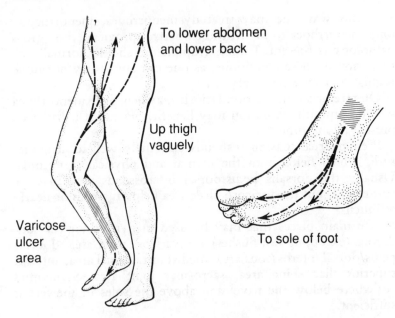

Fig. 8.2 Radiation from varicose ulcer area

The radiation in the sole would fit in with the medial and lateral plantar nerves and artery and with branches of the tibial nerve and posterior tibial artery.

Radiation may also extend upwards, through the thigh to the lower abdomen and lower back.

Diseases and symptoms which may be treated

Abdomen and back

In Chinese tradition, virtually all gynaecological diseases in the lower abdomen may be treated by stimulating spleen 6, provided they are the type of reversible condition amenable to acupuncture. In my experience it does not matter if spleen 6 itself (where a varicose ulcer occurs) or anywhere in the varicose ulcer area is stimulated.

In this way one may treat dysmenorrhoea, menorrhagia, oligomenorrhoea and Mittleschmertz, provided no gross pathology is present. I think acupuncture should normally be tried first in these conditions, as one can always try hormone regulation later if necessary.

On rare occasions, endometriosis may benefit. Amenorrhoea of a few months' duration may benefit, but not if it has been present a long time.

Premenstrual tension responds extremely well to acupuncture, which helps both the mental and physical symptoms. Usually the dorsalis pedis/dorsal interosseous area may be stimulated, but the varicose ulcer area helps as much or nearly as much.

The main places that may be used in gynaecological conditions (excepting hot flushes) are: varicose ulcer area, dorsalis pedis/dorsal interosseous area, medial infragenual area, anterior superior iliac spine area, sacro-iliac joint area. Sometimes anywhere below the navel and above the soles of the feet is sufficient.

Case history. A patient had menorrhagia which occurred every 3 weeks, causing her to be exhausted and inhibiting any activity during the relevant period. A gynaecologist found no gross pathology present and she was not anaemic. Treatment at the varicose ulcer area cured both her menorrhagia and the rather too frequent periods.

Lower leg

As mentioned above, the radiation from the varicose ulcer area may go down the lower leg, probably more frequently medioposteriorly, to the whole sole of the foot and possibly other areas of the foot. Vague aches and pains all along the course of this radiation area may be helped; possibly also mild circulatory dysfunction.

Section 9

CARDIAC AREAS

MEDIAL ARM AREA
Heart 2 to 8; H2 to 8; HT2 to 8

STERNUM
Conception vessel 16 to 22; Cv16 to 22; CV16 to 22

The heart in Chinese medicine is a much wider and vaguer concept than in Western medicine. In this section I will describe ideas which are a mixture of Chinese, Western and my own.

If a patient has angina pectoris, he may have pain or discomfort anywhere in the front or back of the chest, epigastrium, throat, neck, jaw or occiput. In addition there is pain anywhere in either arm.

On examining such a patient one does not, as a rule, find tenderness over the whole area described above. Two areas seem to have a predilection for becoming tender, though on occasion anywhere may do so. I have called these two areas the medial arm area and the sternal area or sternum.

MEDIAL ARM AREA (Fig. 9.1a, b)

The medial arm area extends from the neck of the humerus to the head of the 5th metacarpal and, possibly, beyond, to include the 5th finger.

If the flesh is pressed against the bone, there is tenderness in the upper part of its course corresponding with the antero-medial surface of the humerus, which lies between the anterior and medial borders. This distribution stops at the proximal border of the elbow joint.

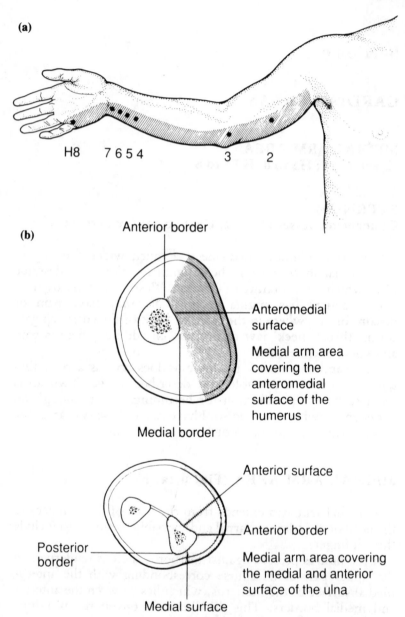

Fig. 9.1 (a) Heart points 2–8. (b) Medial arm area

From the proximal border of the elbow joint to the head of the 5th metacarpal, the area of tenderness on pressure is displaced a little anteriorly, so that it corresponds with the medial and anterior surfaces of the ulna, between the posterior and anterior borders and anterior and interosseous borders respectively. The tenderness of the medial arm area in the elbow and palm corresponds with the anterior displacement along the length of the ulna just described and shown in Fig. 9.1b.

It is possible that the position of the medial arm area is at least partially determined by the neurovascular bundle that runs along almost its entire length, for there is often an enhanced tenderness on pressure over nerves, arteries and veins. In the upper arm are the ulnar nerve, the median nerve, the brachial artery and vein; in the lower arm the ulnar nerve, the ulnar artery and companion vein.

It is interesting that the medial arm area largely corresponds with the course of the Chinese heart meridian and the acupuncture points on it. However, the meridian and points are exceedingly small. In traditional acupuncture the small intestine and heart meridians and their corresponding acupuncture points are 'coupled', so that one may be used instead of the other. It is apparent from my description of the medial arm area that the course of the small intestine meridian is a little posterior to the posterior edge of the medial arm area and hence the 'coupled' link mentioned above does not apply, at least from this point of view. Although much of what I write contradicts or partially contradicts acupuncture tradition, there is, in this section, a considerably greater degree of agreement.

For the purposes of treatment, the medial arm area may be subdivided as follows:

1 ANTERIOR MEDIAL ELBOW AREA (Fig. 9.2)

The patient's arm should be in the anatomical position and, in so far as it is possible, hyperextended. In the majority of people, the whole of the medial half of the anterior surface of the elbow, an area about 5 cm in diameter, consisting of the

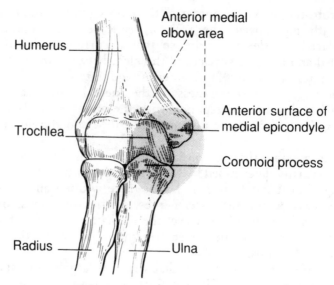

Fig. 9.2 Anterior medial elbow area

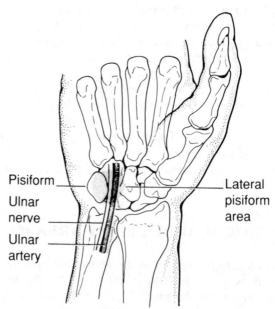

Fig. 9.3 Lateral pisiform area

anterior aspects of the medial epicondyle, the trochlea and coronoid process, is tender. The brachial artery is lateral to this area. The radiation from this area does not fit in with the course of the median nerve. Sometimes the whole of this area is tender, sometimes certain parts, or certain parts are more tender within the whole tender area. The most tender part is needled subcutaneously, intramuscularly or, if stronger stimulation is required, periosteally.

It is interesting that, in some people, this whole area becomes oedematous, as in the medial infragenual area, though to a lesser extent. Anatomically both areas are in nearly equivalent positions.

Acupuncture point heart 3, depending on how it is defined, is within this area.

2 LATERAL PISIFORM AREA (Fig. 9.3)

This area is on the anterior surface of the wrist. It is centred on the pisiform bone with a tender area 2–3 cm in diameter. The place which is most frequently tender is immediately lateral to the pisiform, so that the needle as it enters the deeper tissues just scrapes the lateral side of the pisiform. I do not know if it is significant that the ulnar nerve and artery are in exactly the same position, just lateral to the pisiform.

Acupuncture point heart 7 is within the lateral pisiform area. The usual definition of the point is not the same as my point of maximal tenderness along the lateral side of the pisiform.

STERNUM (Fig. 9.4)

Another important area, where tenderness to pressure may occur in cardiac and pulmonary disease, is the body of the sternum. This tenderness may occur anywhere on the body of the sternum, but is, I think, more marked in the midline. Tenderness may also occur over the manubrium and xiphoid process, but possibly less often. It is interesting that there are five acupuncture points in this area: the upper and lower

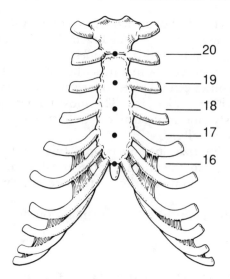

Fig. 9.4 Conception vessel points 16 to 20

correspond with the manubriosternal joint and xiphisternal joint, whereas the middle three correspond with the junctions of the four developmental segments, the sternebrae.

As aforesaid, there are many areas in the upper half of the body which may become tender in cardiac disease but the two referred to above are probably the most frequent.

Radiation

Anterior medial elbow arm and lateral pisiform area (Fig. 9.5)

The radiation from the medial arm area may go anywhere in the arm, chest, upper abdomen, shoulder, neck, face and head.

There is a tendency, but only a tendency, for the radiation from the anterior medial elbow area to go mainly to the chest, the lower half of the neck and, to a lesser extent, the upper abdomen. The radiation is often diffuse, so that the patient can only say he has a sensation in this or that area, without being able to indicate a path from the needle prick to, say, the chest.

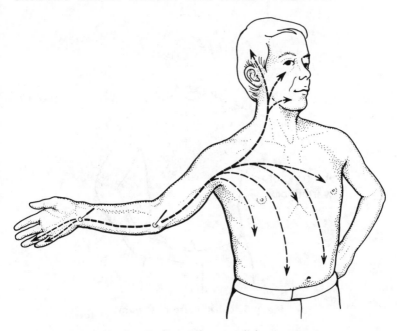

Fig. 9.5 Radiation from medial arm area

The radiation from the lateral pisiform area may go to the same places as that from the anterior medial elbow area, but also goes more often than the latter up the lateral side of the neck to the jaw, face and occiput.

Radiation from anywhere in the medial arm area may go down the medial border of the arm to the 5th and 4th fingers. Sometimes though, it goes to the thumb, lateral or posterior side of the elbow, or the lateral side of the shoulder joint.

Sternum (Fig. 9.6)

Radiation from the sternum is usually confined to the chest. The patient may notice a feeling of warmth, the size of a plate, in the front of the chest, at the back of the chest or within the chest. There are no actual lines of radiation, just a feeling of warmth, or sometimes of cool fresh air.

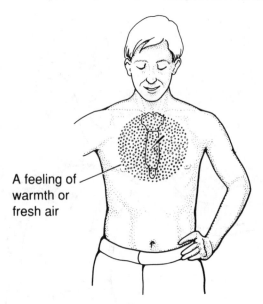

A feeling of
warmth or
fresh air

Fig. 9.6 Radiation from sternum

Diseases and symptoms which may be treated

Cardiac

Mild cardiac conditions may sometimes be treated; severe ones not.

Palpitations constitute a real symptom as far as patients are concerned, even though cardiologists often dismiss them as subjective, the mere somatisation of stress.

Case history. A patient had palpitations which were so severe that she could not ride a bicycle up a hill. I asked her to see a cardiologist, who found nothing objective wrong and thought she was neurotic.

I treated her by acupuncture, first at the lateral pisiform area, then at the anterior medial elbow area. On each occasion the palpitations stopped at once and she was able to ride a bicycle uphill. On each occasion, however, the benefit only lasted 3 days. In acupuncture the benefit of treatment should last longer with each subsequent treatment and, if this does not happen, the doctor must look for other factors that influence the disease or symptoms.

This patient was an art teacher at an unruly school, the children being even more badly behaved during art classes, art not being an examination subject. In the end the patient left the school and started teaching art at an adult education college, where the students wished to learn. Her palpitations and breathlessness on cycling uphill were reduced. I then repeated the acupuncture and she was cured. Obviously the stress was originally so great that acupuncture worked only temporarily. If the stress had been milder, acupuncture would have cured her initially.

The teacher who took over the patient's job at the school of recalcitrant children died from a coronary 6 months later.

Mild angina pectoris, patients who are unduly breathless on exertion, some forms of hyperhidrosis may, where appropriate, respond.

Arrhythmias may respond to needling the sternum, but I normally prefer not to treat such patients. Acupuncture does not help, or if so, only marginally, in congestive cardiac failure or cardiomyopathy. On one occasion, however, I had a patient with a valvular defect who could only walk 1 mile, whereas after acupuncture he would walk 30 miles with less exhaustion. I was nonplussed.

Anxiety

Mild mental states (not real diseases) are, from my point of view, quite often the mental expression of a mild physiological dysfunction. Hence a medical treatment is more appropriate than psychotherapy.

I have several patients with mild asthma who benefit from salbutamol inhalation. Some of these patients notice that after the inhalation their asthma improves but they develop a mild tachycardia. Together with the tachycardia they become anxious. They have no reason to be anxious, given that their asthma is better. They recognise that their anxiety does not have a mental cause and is, in fact, a symptom of the tachycardia.

There are, I think, many people, who do not have a cardiac disease but merely some mild physiological dysfunction, who become *anxious* extremely easily, sometimes for no reason or sometimes for an inadequate reason. These patients are quite often recognised by their manner of speech: they speak almost as if the words cannot tumble out fast enough. Some doctors who have had tachycardia, cardiac arrhythmias or taken a sympathomimetic may recognise this phenomenon from personal experience.

Case history. A patient of 65 had wished her whole life long to go into politics. Unfortunately, however, whenever she spoke in public she felt her 'heart pounding away in her chest'; this was accompanied by such a degree of anxiety that she could not continue. She had to give up what she felt was her vocation.

Treatment at the lateral pisiform area helped her considerably, but did not quite cure her. Unfortunately by then she was too old to fulfil her lifelong ambition.

General symptoms

Any symptoms within the area of radiation mentioned in the previous section may be treated. This includes, as a possibility, anything between the top of the head and the navel. Needless to say, treating this area is not always the best option in all conditions: quite often other treatments may be more appropriate. As always, the doctor must use his judgement and experience.

Mild asthma, being 'chesty' (but not a real infection) may respond. An irreversible pathology such as emphysema is not helped unless there is also spasm, in which case the spasm component may be alleviated. Some patients with chronic chests may be partially helped between courses of antibiotics.

Sometimes pain in the neck, face and head are helped.

Case history. A Bantu patient from South Africa was always a little chesty, presumably due to the cool, damp climate here. Needling the sternum helped, but did not cure him.

Section 10

TRAPEZIUS/OCCIPUT AREA
2 cm from gall bladder 20; G20; GB20

This is one of those areas which is tender in perhaps half the population, though it is more tender in those with headaches or cervical disease (Fig. 10.1a, b).

The patient should be examined sitting in a chair with his hands resting on his lap, so that the nuchal muscles exert some tension to hold the head upright. If the patient lies down, with the nuchal muscles relaxed, it is more difficult to find the area of tenderness.

The tender area is most frequently found where the lateral fibres of the trapezius are attached to the occiput at the superior nuchal line. On a few occasions, the area of the lateral fibres is not tender; one may instead find tenderness where the medial or the intermediate fibres of the trapezius are attached to the occiput (Fig. 10.1a, b). The area of tenderness may be 1–3 cm in diameter. Rarely, there may be tenderness in the upper 5 cm of the trapezius.

If one wishes to stimulate gently, one merely needles the skin or muscle of the tender area. If stronger stimulation is required, the periosteum of the occiput is stimulated and pecked gently or strongly, according to the case.

The greater occipital nerve (dorsal ramus of C2) and occipital artery are near the lateral trapezius/occiput area. The lesser occipital nerve (ventral ramus of C2) is not far away. The 3rd occipital nerve (dorsal ramus of C3) is near the medial or intermediate trapezius/occiput areas.

The trapezius/occiput area may be tender in any disease of the head above the level of the mouth; likewise in patients with symptoms in the neck, throat and shoulders (Fig. 10.2). Although the area of the lower jaw is rarely influenced by needling the trapezius/occiput area, the temporomandibular joint, perhaps surprisingly, may be influenced. As with everything in acupuncture, little is accurate, much is vague and most

(a)

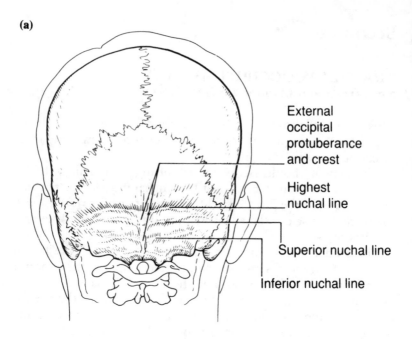

External occipital protuberance and crest

Highest nuchal line

Superior nuchal line

Inferior nuchal line

(b)

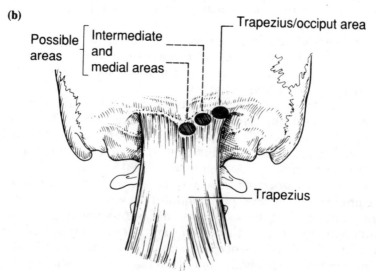

Possible areas

Intermediate and medial areas

Trapezius/occiput area

Trapezius

Fig. 10.1 (a), (b) Trapezius/occiput area

is contradictory: pragmatism takes preference to supposed fact or theory.

Radiation

Radiation is relatively infrequent when needling the trapezius/occiput area. If it does occur, it usually goes over the top of the scalp to the forehead, though occasionally it may go anywhere (Fig. 10.2).

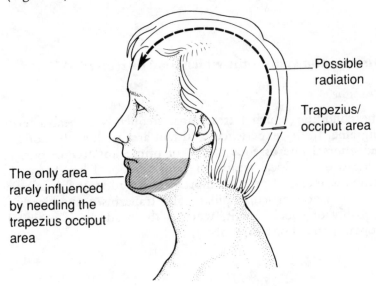

Fig. 10.2 Radiation from trapezius/occiput area

This radiation perhaps fits in with the course of the greater occipital nerve and 3rd occipital nerve on the one hand and of the supraorbital nerve and supratrochlear nerve on the other hand. It may be that a few microscopic fibres of the greater and 3rd occipital nerves extend to the forehead. Perhaps it is related to the course of the occipital, supraorbital and supratrochlear arteries. It is also possible that it is not related to any of these structures.

There is a well-known traditional acupuncture point, gall bladder 20, some 2 cm below and lateral to the trapezius/ occiput area. Gall bladder 20 is below the occiput, lateral to the trapezius and posterior to the sternomastoid. I find that gall bladder 20 is less frequently tender than the trapezius/occiput area, which correlates with my finding that the latter area is more often effective than gall bladder 20, even though occasionally I do find that the reverse is true.

Diseases and symptoms which may be treated

Headache

The condition which I treat most frequently is headache or migraine. In my experience, a distant area such as the dorsalis pedis/dorsal interosseous area is of prime importance but, in some patients, local treatment is of additional benefit or, in some instances, of prime importance. An additional local area is the cervical articular pillar. The trapezius/occiput area is probably of equal benefit, whether the headache is occipital, frontal, parietal or temporal.

Sinus

The trapezius/occiput area may help in frontal or maxillary sinus infection, possibly of the ethmoidal or sphenoidal sinuses also. There are many patients where it is difficult to decide if they have sinus trouble or ordinary headaches. As the treatment of both conditions, from an acupuncture point of view, is much the same, the treatment is straightforward.

Case history. A patient from Ireland had frontal headaches, lasting at least half of every day, which she had had for several years. An X-ray taken previously showed clouding, whereas a recent one did not. Treatment at the trapezius/occiput area and also the dorsalis pedis/ dorsal interosseous area cured her.

Eye

Retro-orbital pain and periorbital pain, such as is seen both by general practitioners and ophthalmologists, responds to the same treatment.

Face

Atypical facial neuralgia may also respond. I think acupuncture is of only marginal use in genuine trigeminal neuralgia: it may help if the area of pain is small and relatively mild and if the patient is a Strong Reactor.

Pain in the face below the level of the lips, I think rarely responds. This naturally includes most of the lower jaw though, interestingly enough, pain in the temporomandibular joint may respond.

I often hear lectures by doctors, and once even by a professor, that acupuncture helps or cures Bell's palsy. About 80% of patients with Bell's palsy recover without any treatment. There is also no disease, as far as I know, where acupuncture helps or cures more than 80% of patients. Hence how one can distinguish one from the other is beyond my comprehension. Perhaps a neurologist with a particularly extensive experience of Bell's palsy might know. If a patient has already had Bell's palsy for a year and natural recovery has ceased, I doubt if acupuncture helps. It has done so on one exceptional occasion, where I used scalp acupuncture.

There is a rare form of facial palsy, mimicking Bell's palsy, which is really a symptom of migraine and responds well to migraine treatment. Pain in an upper canine, identical to toothache, may also be the only symptom of migraine, and thus responds likewise to migraine treatment.

Case history. The son of a dentist (it would be) had pain in an upper canine and nowhere else. X-rays and other tests revealed nothing. Treatment at the dorsalis pedis/dorsal interosseous area and at the trapezius/occiput area cured him.

Neck

Pain in the neck is generally best treated by needling the cervical articular pillar but sometimes, particularly if the referred pain is in the face, the trapezius/occiput area is better.

Case history. A patient had pain at the back of the neck on the right. She also had pain at the top of her head on the left. The major pain, however, was at the root of the nose on both sides. Treatment at the trapezius/occiput area cured her.

Peculiar pains and a feeling of constriction in the throat respond to the same treatment.

The principal doctor, whose clinics I attended when at the hospital in Peking (Beijing), was a specialist in gall bladder 20 which, although it is some 2 or 2.5 cm from my area, has much the same effect. He treated many eye diseases and patients were referred to him specifically when it was considered that this point was the most important one in the treatment.

Section 11

MASTOID PROCESS AREA
Roughly gall bladder 12; G12; GB12

Patients who have headache, neck pain or pain in the face should be examined at the base of the skull, from one mastoid process right round to the other mastoid process. The most frequent tender area is the lateral trapezius/occiput area. In some patients though, the region of the mastoid process is tender, particularly the posterior and inferior aspect, near the attachment of the sternomastoid (Fig. 11.1).

The most tender area, which is usually posterior or inferior to the mastoid process, is palpated. Then the needle is inclined in whatever direction is required to needle the periosteum of the posterior or inferior pole of the mastoid process: i.e. anteromedially or superomedially, respectively.

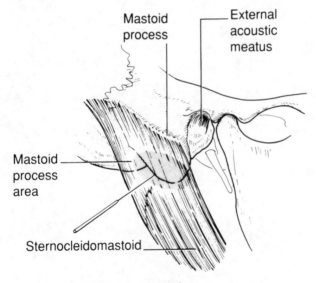

Fig. 11.1 Mastoid process area

The effect of needling is noticed mainly in the lower half of the skull, posterior to the external acoustic meatus. This is a place I do not use frequently.

Section 12

LAMBDOID SUTURE AREA
Possibly gall bladder 19; G19; GB19

Sometimes there is a tender area, very roughly 4 cm above and lateral to the lateral trapezius/occiput area (Fig. 12.1). It usually corresponds with a slight indentation of the skull, which I think corresponds with the lambdoid suture. Possibly gall bladder 19 fits in with this area, though it is difficult to know as the position of the Chinese point is defined by geometry not anatomy.

The lambdoid suture area may be needled in conditions similar to those in which one uses the trapezius/occiput area. It is a place I rarely use.

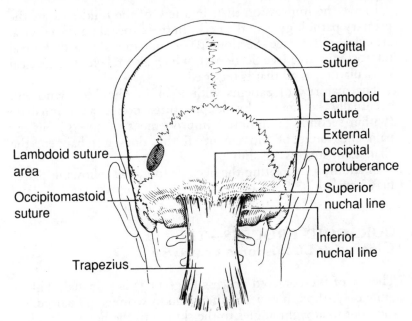

Fig. 12.1 Lambdoid suture area

Section 13

PAINFUL SHOULDER

Acupuncture, in my experience at least, will help a painful shoulder in a moderate proportion of patients, provided the range of movement is full or nearly full. I think it only helps a moderate proportion, though there are some doctors who can cure a higher proportion than I can and, what is more, can even help those patients who have moderately severe or sometimes even severe restriction of movement, i.e. a frozen shoulder. Possibly these doctors are treating acute cases, whereas in my practice I see virtually exclusively only chronic cases. Osteoarthritis of the glenohumeral joint is, in my experience, helped only temporarily; the same is true of calcification of the supraspinatus tendon.

I have the impression that, in a few of the milder cases, the primary pathology is in the neck. In these, needling the cervical articular pillar (see Section 4) or the dorsalis pedis/dorsal interosseous area (see Section 5), which also relaxes the cervical musculature, is all that is required.

The majority of patients with a painful shoulder, who will eventually be helped by acupuncture, notice an immediate (within seconds or minutes) improvement of 50–75% in the pain and range of movement. If this does not happen, the chances of success are slim.

In addition to treating the neck or foot, the following places may be tried.

CORACOID PROCESS—TIP
Lung 1; L1; LU1; is some 3 cm away

The tip of the coracoid process (Fig. 13.1) is palpated. This is quite easy, though easier in men than in women. The needle is then put in at right angles to the skin until the bone is touched and then lightly pecked, as is usual in periosteal acupuncture.

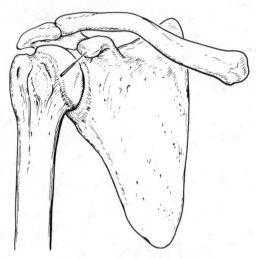

Fig. 13.1 Coracoid process

Radiation

Radiation from the tip of the coracoid process is less frequent than in the majority of areas mentioned until now in this book. It may, however, occur (Fig. 13.2) to:

The upper lateral quadrant of the chest wall.
The upper two-thirds of the upper arm. It is usually felt inside the arm, rather than on the surface.
The whole area of the scapula.
Across the top of the shoulder and up the posterolateral aspect of the neck.

INFRASPINATUS AREAS
Hansen I Area
Small intestine 11; Si11; SI11

The patient should be sitting in a chair with his arms at his side.

The Hansen I area is 2 or 3 cm below the medial third of the

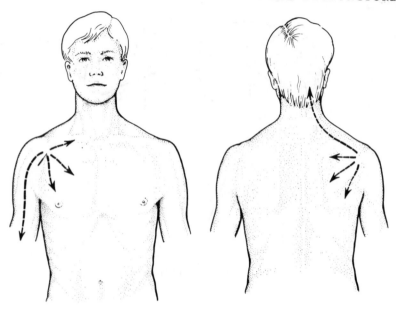

Fig. 13.2 Radiation from tip of coracoid process

spine of the scapula in the trapezius. Needling this area peri-
osteally usually achieves the best result. Radiation from the
Hansen I area may go to the shoulder and down the whole arm
(Fig. 13.3).

The traditional acupuncture point, small intestine 11, is
several centimetres lateral to Hansen I. It is lateral to the
trapezius, medial to the deltoid and just below the apex of the
inverted V where their tendinous areas cross one another.
Radiation from small intestine 11 usually goes only to the
shoulder.

Usually, Hansen I is more effective than small intestine 11.

Dr Peer Walther Hansen of Copenhagen discovered this area,
which I have therefore called Hansen I.

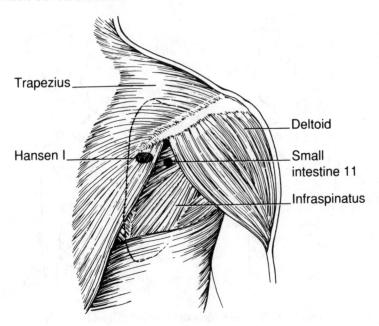

Fig. 13.3 Infraspinatus areas

INFRAGLENOID TUBERCLE
Hansen II. Does not correspond with any standard acupuncture point

Needling the infraglenoid tubercle, to which the long head of the triceps is attached, helps some patients with a painful shoulder.

The arm should be held as shown in Fig. 13.4, with the fingers around the back of the opposite shoulder. The infraglenoid tubercle can be identified easily only in the slimmer patient and hence I do not think it advisable to use this technique in those who are overweight. The teres minor, followed by the long head of the triceps, are stimulated before the infraglenoid tubercle is reached.

Radiation from the infraglenoid tubercle may go to the lower arm.

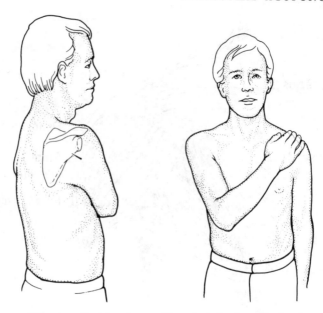

Fig. 13.4 Position for needling the infraglenoid tubercle

This tender area was also discovered by Dr Peer Walther Hansen of Copenhagen and it is therefore called Hansen II.

Some patients with a painful shoulder are also helped by exercises, but others are not or may even be made worse.

In my experience, rest is more often of benefit. I ask the patient:

1 Not to do any movement which hurts, which usually means upwards and backwards, though it does vary from individual to individual.
2 Not to do any similar movement, even if it does not hurt.

I have found that the wrong movement, only once a day, is enough to inhibit healing. The rest–cure approach to a painful shoulder thus requires single-minded dedication, entailing as it does a change in how one does even the most routine movements, i.e. opening sash windows, combing one's hair, etc.

Section 14

THE FOOT
METATARSOPHALANGEAL REGION

There are many, particularly elderly, patients who have pain in this region. It occurs in those who have deformed toes associated with rheumatoid arthritis; in those who have a deformity in another part of the foot causing undue strain on the transverse arch; and, of course, on the medial side in those with a bunion or osteoarthritis of the 1st metatarsophalangeal joint. There are also those who have pain over the head of one metatarsal only, restricted to the plantar side.

JUNCTION OF HEAD AND SHAFT OF METATARSAL 1 or 5
Spleen 3; Sp3; SP3 or bladder 65; B65; BL65

HEAD OF METATARSAL
Does not correspond with any standard acupuncture point

If the pain is restricted to the region of the first joint, the junction of the head and shaft of the first metatarsal may be needled (Fig. 14.1). The needle pierces the soft tissues at the junction of the head and shaft of the 1st metatarsal on the plantar side. If the foot is in the normal position on the ground (it is in practice probably on the doctor's lap), the needle is put in from medial to lateral, parallel to the floor. The depth of needling may be varied: one may stimulate the periosteum on the medial side of the junction of the head and shaft of the 1st metatarsal; however, I usually stimulate the angle between the head and shaft on the plantar side, as shown in Fig. 14.1.

If, more unusually, the pain is restricted to the lateral side of this transverse arch, the treatment is exactly the same as that

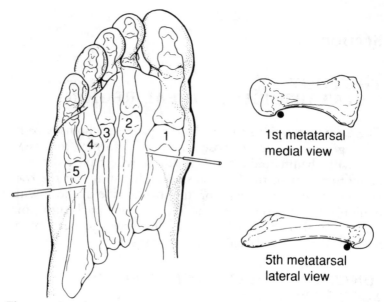

1st metatarsal
medial view

5th metatarsal
lateral view

Fig. 14.1 Junction of head and shaft of metatarsals 1 and 5, with needles in plantar position

mentioned above, except that the junction of the head and shaft on the plantar side of the 5th metatarsal is stimulated, the needle being inserted from lateral to medial.

If the whole of the transverse arch is painful, the junctions of the head and shaft on the plantar side of both the 1st and 5th metatarsals are stimulated.

Sometimes there is pain over the head of one metatarsal only, restricted to the plantar side and normally occurring only in heads 2, 3 or 4. In these patients, the heads of the metatarsals are palpated from the plantar side to ascertain which is the tender head; this is not always easy. After very careful localisation of the most tender area, the needle is inserted through the sole of the foot to stimulate the relevant metatarsal head on the plantar side—a painful procedure. Sometimes the junction of the head and shaft of the 1st and 5th metatarsals may be stimulated in addition, as described above: the 1st from the medial side, the 5th from the lateral side.

As mentioned in Section 15, treatment of the equivalent area in the hand, i.e. the knuckles, is the same, involving stimulation of the junction of the head and shaft of the metacarpals.

ANTERIOR TUBERCLE OF CALCANEUS
MEDIAL AND LATERAL PROCESS OF
CALCANEAL TUBEROSITY
Neither correspond to a standard acupuncture point

Plantar fasciitis

The gastrocnemius tendon area, described in detail in Section 7, is the treatment of first choice.

Sometimes in patients with plantar fasciitis I needle the tender area directly. This is usually situated in the region of the anterior tubercle on the plantar surface of the calcaneus (Fig. 14.2). Using a 23-gauge hypodermic needle, I go through the

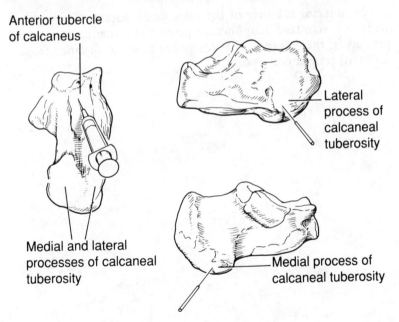

Fig. 14.2 Treatment of plantar fasciitis

skin of the heel on the plantar side, infiltrate the tender area with 0.5–1.00 ml of local anaesthetic and then peck the periosteum. I use this technique because the pecking of a dry acupuncture needle in this area would be more painful. I ask the patient to walk as little as possible for the remainder of the day. One should note that overstrong stimulation may easily aggravate the pain. As an alternative, the medial process of the calcaneal tuberosity may be needled from the medial side and the lateral process of the calcaneal tuberosity may be needled from the lateral side (Fig. 14.2).

Case history. A patient had pain in his heel with every step. There was a hard, tender, indurated area half the size of a broad bean in the region of the anterior tubercle of the calcaneus, something I had not noted previously with other patients. Gentle and then somewhat stronger needling at the gastrocnemius tendon area helped only for 1 hour. Local anaesthetic and pecking of the anterior tubercle of the calcaneous caused him agony for 2 days and some worsening for 2 weeks. Nothing I could do helped him.

The anterior tubercle of the calcaneous does not correspond with any standard acupuncture point. The medial and lateral process of the calcaneal tuberosity are at some distance from a standard acupuncture point.

Section 15

THE HAND AND WRIST

There are many diseases of the wrist and hand which cause pain, swelling or restriction of movement. Among them are rheumatoid arthritis, osteoarthritis and Dupuytren's contracture. As mentioned previously, acupuncture may help mild osteoarthritis, mild burnt-out rheumatoid arthritis, seronegative arthritides or the earliest stage of Dupuytren's contracture. It rarely helps inactive rheumatoid arthritis, advanced osteoarthritis or tenosynovitis.

General treatment

Needling the cervical articular pillar (see Section 4) has a general effect on the whole arm. If a patient has a disease or symptom *anywhere* in the arm which is *mild* and, preferably, the patient is a *Strong Reactor*, needling the neck may help. It can on occasion be amazing how the mere needling of the cervical articular pillar may cure or alleviate virtually anything in the arm of *an appropriate patient*.

A similar general effect on the medial side of the arm and hand may be achieved by needling the anterior medial elbow area (trochlea, coronoid process, medial epicondyle) (see Section 9). The lateral side of the arm and hand may be influenced by needling the anterior lateral elbow area (head of radius, capitulum, lateral epicondyle) from anteriorly (see Section 17).

LATERAL WRIST AREA
Large intestine 5; Li5; LI5

Pain, some limitation of movement and a moderate degree of swelling may occur in a burnt-out rheumatoid or in the

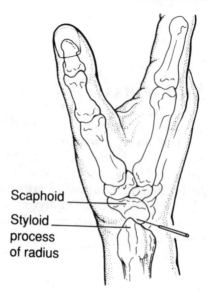

Fig. 15.1 Lateral wrist area

seronegative arthritides. These may be helped to a limited extent. The commonest site of symptoms is on the lateral and medial side of the wrist.

On the lateral side of the wrist the symptoms occur in the anatomical snuff box between the lower end of the radius and the small carpal bones (scaphoid). The needle is inserted (Fig. 15.1) from lateral to medial at the level of the tip of the styloid process of the radius. One may needle the tip of the styloid process or penetrate 1 or 2 mm posteriorly. The lateral wrist area corresponds to large intestine 5.

MEDIAL WRIST AREA
Probably small intestine 5; Si5; SI5

On the medial side of the wrist, pain or tenderness most frequently occurs between the lower end of the ulna and the small wrist bone (triquetral). The needle is inserted 1 or 2 mm

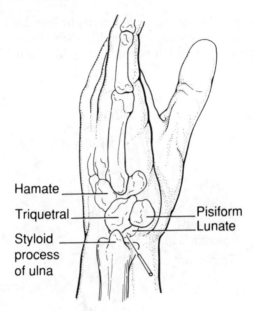

Fig. 15.2 Medial wrist area

proximal and anterior to the tip of the styloid process of the ulna (Fig. 15.2). The medial wrist area probably corresponds with small intestine 5, though some authors place the Chinese point 2 cm distal, on the pisiform.

1st CARPOMETACARPAL JOINT
Does not correspond with any standard acupuncture point

Pain associated with osteoarthritis often develops in the 1st carpometacarpal joint, preventing patients from gripping objects firmly between the thumb and other fingers.

The joint should be examined carefully. Firm pressure usually elicits a tender area the size of a small pea which is further medial than one might expect. It is about 2 cm medial to the junction of the hairless with the hairy skin. If the radial artery at the wrist were to continue in a straight line distally, it would cross this area, which coincides with a small unnamed osseous protruberance, one which is tender also in a healthy hand (Fig. 15.3).

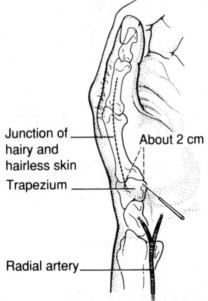

Fig. 15.3 1st carpometacarpal joint

The 1st carpometacarpal joint area does not correspond with any standard acupuncture point. Lung 10 is 1 or 2 cm further distal along the shaft of the 1st metacarpal.

This tender area is painful and should be needled with care. If the needling is gentle, it may work in one patient and fail in another. If it is done too strongly, the patient may have to be scraped off the ceiling and will then curse you for 2 days, after which there may or may not be an improvement.

General treatment

Stimulation of the cervical articular pillar helps mild cases.

Needling the anterior lateral elbow area (see Section 17) may help others.

Needling anywhere on the anterior or lateral surface of the radius may help; however, it is possible that needling the anterior lateral elbow area, which is more tender in most patients, is of greater benefit. Points such as this, which are tender on pressure in most people, whether or not they have a disease, are usually more effective.

It is such observations, which can be repeated time and again, which cast serious doubt on the existence of acupuncture points, as traditionally conceived.

This treatment helps the milder cases, but rarely the more severe ones.

JUNCTION OF HEAD AND SHAFT OF METACARPAL 2 or 5
Large intestine 3; Li3; LI3; or small intestine 3; Si3; SI3

The knuckles may be affected in rheumatoid arthritis. The pain, swelling and limitation of movement may be partially alleviated in a mild, burnt-out rheumatoid patient. It may also help a patient with seronegative rheumatoid arthritis.

The treatment is essentially similar to the treatment of symptoms in the metatarsophalangeal joints described in Section 14.

If, as sometimes occurs, the symptoms are restricted to the 2nd metacarpophalangeal joint, the junction of the head and shaft of the 2nd metacarpal is needled. The needle is inserted from lateral to medial, in the angle between the head and shaft on the palmar side, as shown in Fig. 15.4.

If all the knuckles are affected, the 5th metacarpal is needled as well, though in this instance, of course, the needle is inserted from medial to lateral. The point of insertion is roughly where the skin with hair becomes hairless.

Heberden's nodes

These may be treated by acupuncture at an early stage of their development, when they consist of a gelatinous swelling. Later,

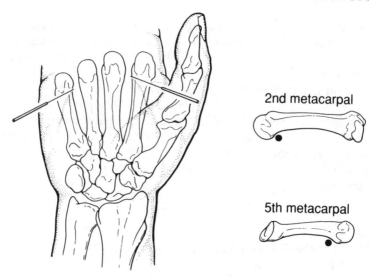

Fig. 15.4 Junction of head and shaft of metacarpal 2 or 5, palmar aspect

when they become ossified, treatment does not help except, perhaps, marginally.

The patient's hand is put flat, palm down on a table and, as the procedure is painful, the hand must be held tightly. Each Heberden's node is pierced down to the bone which, if all fingers are affected, means 20 painful pricks. The treatment is repeated a few times at, say, fortnightly intervals.

Frequently the gelatinous swellings reduce in size by, say, some 50% and the pain stops. What is more important is that the soft swelling does not become ossified. I think that the large hard swellings and deformity of the distal interphalangeal joint can thus often be avoided or partially avoided.

Dupuytren's contracture

This may be treated at a very early stage of the disease, when only one or two nodules, smaller than a split lentil, are present and when there is no flexion deformity whatsoever. Once the nodules are more numerous, larger and there is flexion of a finger or additional creases in the palm, the situation is hopeless and it is not even worth trying acupuncture.

The patient's hand is put on a table, palm upwards. As this procedure is painful the hand must be held tightly. The one or two nodules in the palmar fascia are isolated carefully and needled, the needle piercing the skin at right angles. This is repeated a few times at, say, fortnightly intervals.

I then ask the patient to stimulate the nodule himself, using a blunt pointed instrument, such as the tip of a deer's antler, or the top of the currently produced Bic ball-point pen. The instrument is applied to the skin until it hurts. The patient must do this initially once a day, then on alternate days, twice a week, once a week, until the nodules are about half their previous size. If the instrument is too sharp it will cut into the patient's hand; if it is too blunt, the pressure will be dispersed over too large an area.

Section 16

THE VERTEBRAL COLUMN

SPINOUS PROCESS
INTERSPINOUS LIGAMENT
SACROSPINALIS—ERECTOR SPINAE

The neck has been discussed in Section 4. The most important local area of stimulation is the cervical articular pillar, though one may also needle the trapezius/occiput area. Often distant needling is of greater benefit, particularly the dorsalis pedis/dorsal interosseus area or, sometimes, the lateral pisiform area.

Lumbar spine

The lumbar spine has also been discussed. I frequently needle the sacro-iliac joint area, the anterior superior iliac spine area, the lumbar spinous processes, the lumbar interspinous ligaments and the lumbar part of the sacrospinalis.

Upper thoracic spine

Interscapular pain is most frequently treated via the neck. It might be remembered that the most frequent radiation observed from needling the cervical articular pillar is interscapular. The radiation runs immediately medial to the medial border of the scapula as far as its inferior angle though, rarely, it may go as far as the lumbar area (see Fig. 4.3). If a patient with interscapular pain does not respond to cervical treatment, treatment as for the lower thoracic spine (see below) may be tried.

Lower thoracic spine

The lower half of the thoracic spine is the most difficult to treat. I understand this concurs with the experience of osteopathic doctors.

Sometimes treatment of both the cervical and lumbar spine will alleviate lower thoracic symptoms.

The thoracic spinous processes may be needled in the midline, with the needle at right angles to the skin (Fig. 16.1).

The thoracic interspinous ligament may also be needled in the midline, with the needle at right angles to the skin (Fig. 16.1).

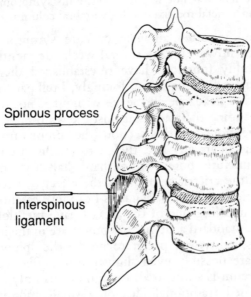

Spinous process

Interspinous ligament

Fig. 16.1 The spinous processes in the thoracic spine point downwards. The spinous processes in the lumbar spine are more horizontal (see Fig. 3.1)

The sacrospinalis on both sides should be palpated as a tender area may often be found on one or other side, usually about 3 cm from the midline. This tender area may be needled.

In ankylosing spondylitis or Scheuermann's disease, all spinous processes, or all interspinous ligaments, or the whole length of both sacrospinalis muscles may be needled, with reasonable results in a small proportion of patients.

Case history. A patient had Scheuermann's disease severely enough to stop him going to school as he could only sit still in a chair for a short while before the pain became unbearable.

Treatment of only the cervical and lumbar spine had no effect. Thereafter the whole of the spine was treated: either the spinous processes or the interspinous ligaments or paravertebrally—all worked equally well. He was able to go back to school for half a day and then full-time.

Some time afterwards, he suddenly decided to go on a 10 kilometre cross-country run (without my knowledge). All the pain returned and further treatment was not able to alleviate his symptoms again. Thereafter he had a metal rod fixed to his vertebral column.

Acupuncture can often alleviate or cure symptoms very quickly. It may, however, take several weeks or months until the various bodily functions have re-established themselves enough to withstand undue strain. Jokingly, I tell patients who arrive here with a headache and leave without it not to test it too much by banging their heads against the wall.

The areas mentioned in this section (the spinous processes, the interspinous ligaments and the sacrospinalis) fit in with standard acupuncture points in perhaps half the instances (depending on the criteria used). Yet the effect of needling a 'correct' acupuncture point is, as far as I can tell, essentially no different from needling one of the areas I have mentioned. In the midline, the standard acupuncture points are in the interspinous ligaments, whereas I prefer to needle the spinous processes, which are possibly even slightly more effective given that the periosteum is stimulated. I mention this only to show that the supposed traditional idea of a small and precisely defined acupuncture point is incorrect, though the general conception of tender areas or reflexly effective non-tender areas is the basis of this book.

Section 17

THE CHEST

STERNUM
Conception vessel 15 to 22; Cv15 to 22; CV15 to 22

ANTERIOR LATERAL ELBOW AREA
Lung 5; L5; LU5

SPINOUS PROCESSES T1 to T9

Chest diseases may be treated by acupuncture to a limited extent. As a rule, orthodox medicine is of primary importance. Only in selected cases may acupuncture be the treatment of first choice; in others it may supplement orthodox medicine; whereas in still others it might be worth trying one or two treatments to see if one has luck. It is possible to do this, as the initial improvement in acupuncture happens quickly if at all.

Diseases and symptoms which may be treated

Asthma

Perhaps 10–20% of patients may be helped to a greater or lesser extent. Only the mild cases respond. Patients who take steroids most of the time very rarely respond. Sometimes there is difficulty in deciding if a patient is just 'chesty' or has asthma: these patients are more likely to respond.

In my experience quite a number (I cannot estimate the proportion) of asthmatics have basically a food allergy. Most frequently this is a sensitivity to milk products, though it may be any substance in food, air or water.

Case history. A patient had an asthmatic cough, mild asthma, hay fever and felt generally not well. Treatment of the liver (see Chapter V) at either the dorsalis pedis/dorsal interosseous area (liver 3) or at the lower chest anteriorly (liver 14) cured her asthmatic cough and asthma and improved her general health.

The improvement lasted some 2 months. The treatment was repeated and again it lasted 2 months. This happened several times; after each single treatment there was 2 months' freedom from symptoms.

If this pattern occurs, it is a sign that the acupuncture is working but that there is also another factor present interfering with the treatment. This can happen in patients who also have a food allergy; in patients with an advanced, irreversible pathology such as cancer or gall stones, where acupuncture can alleviate or cure symptoms always for a specified period of time; or in patients with tachycardia taking thyroxine. In all these instances 'the other factor' has to be dealt with as well.

This patient stopped eating all dairy products. After a month all her symptoms were cured. Whenever she 'sinned' and had some dairy produce, her symptoms returned. She would then return to her diet strictly; this was sometimes enough, though on a few occasions she would need acupuncture as well.

This patient, as aforesaid, also had hay fever during the usual hay fever season. When she cut out all milk products, the hay fever was also cured. It is thus apparent that the primary sensitivity was to milk products, whereas the grass pollen was only a secondary factor. As far as I am aware, not many allergists take such factors into account.

Chronic chests, bronchiectasis, emphysema

Some chronic chest patients with mixed pathology may be helped to a moderate degree. They may be in bed a substantial part of the winter; their chests may sound like clapped out organ pipes; or they may have sarcoidosis. Even if acupuncture helps only a little, the patients think it is worthwhile if they have less dyspnoea, fewer chest infections, feel they can take a deeper breath and feel generally better. I do not know if objective pulmonary function tests are altered.

Pneumonia, acute bronchitis

Should be treated by orthodox medicine.

Tietze's syndrome or costochondritis

May be helped in some patients.

Treatment

A needle anywhere in the front or back of the thorax or anywhere in the arms may help. This, as I frequently repeat in this book, is why I do not believe in the traditional concept of acupuncture points and meridians.

However, as mentioned elsewhere, those areas of the body which are always a little tender in both health and disease are, on the whole, more effective than other areas. The only such tender area in the field under discussion is the anterior lateral elbow area (see below). The manubriosternal joint is possibly more tender than the rest of the sternum. The sternum and spinous processes of the thoracic vertebrae are perhaps more effective than elsewhere, as, in these, the periosteum may be stimulated.

ANTERIOR LATERAL ELBOW AREA
Lung 5; L5; LU5

This consists of the anterior surface of the head of the radius, the capitulum and the lateral epicondyle (Fig. 17.1). It can be felt most easily if the patient tries to hyperextend his elbow with the arm in the anatomical position. The acupuncture point lung 5 is within this area.

Radiation (Fig. 17.2)

The proximal radiation, as far as I can tell, is the same as that from the anterior medial elbow area (see Fig. 9.5). It goes up the arm to the chest and, possibly, upper abdomen bilaterally. It also goes up the neck, head and face ipsilaterally.

Distally the radiation is different, going, as a rule, down the lateral side of the arm to the thumb, though sometimes it does go to the medial side (see Fig. III.4).

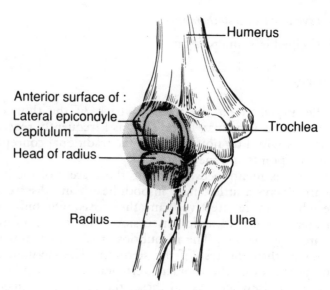

Fig. 17.1 Anterior lateral elbow area

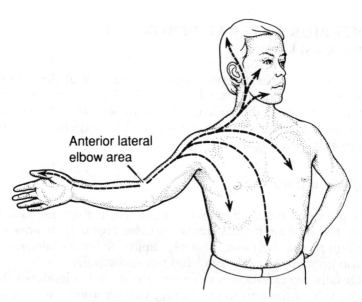

Fig. 17.2 Radiation from anterior lateral elbow area

In traditional acupuncture, the anterior lateral elbow area (lung 5) and other lung acupuncture points on the arm, which are on its anterolateral surface, are supposed to have an effect in pulmonary conditions. As far as I can tell, however, needling anywhere in the arm is equally effective. The two most easily tender areas in the arm, namely the anterior lateral elbow area (lung 5) and the anterior medial elbow area (heart 3) are perhaps the most effective.

Sternum, spinous processes, etc.

The sternum has already been mentioned in Section 9, for it is just as much a heart as a lung area. I sometimes think the manubriosternal joint is slightly more effective. Do remember that the body of the sternum and xiphoid process may have a hole through the middle.

The spinous processes are mentioned in Section 16. In my experience the upper six thoracic spinous processes may be used although, according to Hansen and Schliack, T7 to T10 could also be used.

As mentioned previously, anywhere on the chest will have some effect, including, of course, the classical acupuncture points.

Frequently the upper half of the interscapular area is used.

Tietze's syndrome or costochondritis

If an upper rib is affected and the patient is thin, one can needle the affected rib a few centimetres on either side of the tender nodule. The rib must be palpated very carefully to avoid a pneumothorax. In a fatter person, or if lower ribs are affected, it is dangerous to needle the rib. One may instead prick the skin around the tender nodule in a circle, say 7 cm in diameter. Alternatively, the spinous process, the interspinous ligament or sacrospinalis, in the same segment as the affected rib may be needled. Given that needling of the cervical articular pillar may cause radiation to spread over the anterior chest wall, it is another possible method of treatment.

Section 18

THE FACE

SUPRAORBITAL MARGIN/SUPRATROCHLEAR NERVE AREA
Bladder 2; B2; BL2

INFRAORBITAL FORAMEN AREA
Stomach 2; S2; ST2

Diseases or symptoms in the face can often be treated to advantage by needling distant areas:

1 *Dorsalis pedis/dorsal interosseous area* (see Section 5) may cause radiation in neck, head and face.
2 *Medial arm area* (see Section 9) may cause radiation in neck, head and face.
3 *Lateral elbow area* (see Section 17) may cause radiation in neck, head and face.

The neck and lower occiput are sometimes the cause of facial disease or symptoms and they can also cause radiation to the face:

1 *Cervical articular pillar* (see Section 4) may cause radiation in neck, head and face.
2 *Trapezius/occiput area* (see Section 10) may cause radiation to neck, head and face.

Any of the above five areas may help or cure facial symptoms or disease. In fact the majority of such patients can be treated in this way and only a minority require a needle in the face, as described below.

SUPRAORBITAL MARGIN/SUPRATROCHLEAR NERVE AREA
Bladder 2; B2; BL2

This area, about a centimetre in diameter, is at the supraorbital margin, where it is crossed by the supratrochlear nerve (Fig. 18.1). This is one of the few places in the body where the tender area is always small and in the same position. It is also one of those places which is always tender in both health and disease, though in disease the area may be larger and somewhat more tender.

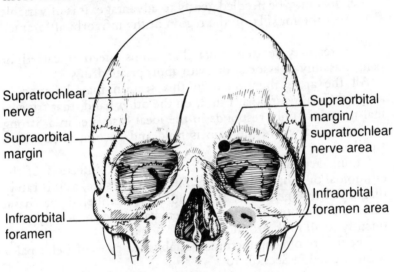

Fig. 18.1 Important areas on the face

Many doctors and patients know this area from their own experience and also know that firm pressure on it—or gentle needlings—may temporarily alleviate a mild headache.

This area may assist in the treatment of a frontal sinus infection.

In some patients with a frontal headache, it is difficult to decide if they have a sinus infection, sinus catarrh or just an ordinary headache. In all instances the supraorbital margin/

supratrochlear nerve area may help. A distant area or the neck may, however, be more effective and, of course, orthodox medical treatment should not be forgotten in acute cases.

INFRAORBITAL FORAMEN AREA
Stomach 2; S2; ST2

Unlike the previously mentioned area, this is an area which is not tender in health. In disease it may or may not become tender. If it is tender, but not if it is exquisitely tender, the tender area may be needled gently to advantage. It is of variable size, over the maxilla, in the region of the infraorbital foramen (Fig. 18.1).

The area may be used in maxillary sinus infection, catarrh or pain, possibly in association with appropriate drugs.

All the areas mentioned in this section may be used in atypical facial neuralgia. I find, on the other hand, that trigeminal neuralgia only responds in the ideal case, i.e. in a Strong Reactor, and where the pain is mild and encompasses only a small area.

I think acupuncture can help in a chronic infection of the ethmoidal or sphenoidal sinuses but I am not sure, as it is rarely diagnosed by specialists. It should be remembered that nasal catarrh and sinus disease are often basically an allergy, frequently to all milk products.

The failure of acupuncture in established cases of Bell's palsy is mentioned in Section 10.

Addendum

Since this book was published in 1992 I have, of course, as is usual in medicine, had new ideas, revised old ideas and, what is often important, changed the emphasis. This change in emphasis is often crucial, as I am increasingly finding that acupuncture is a delicate art where the exact 'dosage' is as important as the place stimulated.

AREAS

The areas which are often the most effective are those which are somewhat tender even in health, but which may become even more tender in disease, such as the gastrocnemius tendon area (p. 139).

The gastrocnemius tendon area may, rarely, be the size of a pea, usually it is the size indicated in Fig. 7.1, but sometimes it may encompass the whole area covered by the gastrocnemius, the soleus and the calcanean tendon. Occasionally the whole leg becomes the 'tender area'. As I have often written, variability is as great as with McBurney's point.

However:

(a) The fingers and toes are rarely tender in disease, yet they are effective in treatment. However, if a tender area can be found, it may well produce a better response.

(b) In a system of Korean hand acupuncture there are 150 acupuncture points on each middle finger, which caused the late Yosio Manaka to wonder if there was any skin left which was not an acupuncture point.

Doctors who practise acupuncture have to learn to live with endless contradictions and apparent inconsistencies.

It should not be forgotten that the 'areas' described in Part II are of course the same whether one uses micro-acupuncture or periosteal acupuncture.

RADIATION

It should again be stressed that the 'radiation' mentioned in all sections of Part II is most easily elicited with periosteal stimulation, particularly in a Strong Reactor. Sometimes one can have radiation with subcutaneous or intramuscular needling, particularly if the needle is manipulated. Radiation occurs less often with micro-acupuncture, except in Hyper-Strong Reactors, though the effect of the micro-acupuncture will be just as great in the appropriate patient.

NEEDLING TECHNIQUE

In recent years the technique I use in periosteal acupuncture has become more gentle. I now, on most occasions, stimulate the periosteum only once and even then extremely gently.

Gradually the way I practise acupuncture in general, whether it be micro-acupuncture or periosteal acupuncture, has become gentler and more frugal, so that quite a high proportion of patients are:

1 *Stimulated in only one place*
2 *The stimulus is gentle. Either micro-acupuncture or gentle periosteal acupuncture.*
3 *The needle remains in place only 1 to 5 seconds.*

If a distant place is needled, such as the foot for a patient with migraine, often gentle micro-acupuncture is sufficient.

If a local area is needled, such as the neck in a patient with migraine, somewhat stronger needling may be required.

Musculo-skeletal conditions, particularly if needled locally, may require gentle periosteal stimulation.

AT WHAT DEPTH ARE THE ACUPUNCTURE AREAS OR POINTS

The tender areas described in this book are of variable size, shape and position and can be felt as tenderness by the patient and, often, as an area of hardness by the doctor's examining fingers. But where are these tender and hard areas, which may be as small as a pea or as large as a whole limb?

For over a century, doctors have found 'fibrositic' nodules in the superficial fascia, without finding anything histologically. Naturally, many acupuncturists equated these with acupuncture points and tried to search for histological structures in this subcutaneous fatty layer.

Others have noticed that these areas may coincide with an area of muscle which feels tender and hard. However, I have shown (in *Textbook of Acupuncture*, pp. 85–6) that the pain and tenderness may disappear without any alteration in the hardness of the muscle and also that there are no electromyographic changes when using surface electrodes.

Subject to further verification, I am inclined to think that what happens in reality is far more extensive, and that the acupuncture area consists of all layers from the epidermis to the periosteum.

This can be verified most easily in a patient who has an unusually extensive tender area:

1 If a tender area is explored where there is no subcutaneous fat and a fold of skin is pulled up between thumb and index finger, and then pinched, one finds that the skin is more tender than a corresponding fold from the other, normal side. On light pressure or stroking, the skin may sometimes also be more

tender than on the normal side. This is why I think that the superficial as well as the deep layers of the skin form part of a 'tender area'.

2 If, in a tender area which has subcutaneous fat, a larger wodge of tissue is taken between the thumb and index finger, to include the fatty layer, one finds that the fatty layer is tender on squeezing. Hence this layer is also part of the 'tender area'.

3 If a tender area is taken with little or no subcutaneous fat and likewise a large fold of tissue is taken to include the muscle, it will be found that the muscle is tender. Hence I include the muscle layer as part of the 'tender area'.

A muscle, particularly the edge of a muscle, is often the only large structure, between the skin and the periosteum, that has any definite shape. Hence, if one presses a tender area, the only structure one feels is a muscle. If the structure of a muscle were as amorphous as that of the subcutaneous fatty layer, one would be, relatively speaking, blind to its existence. Those who place tender areas or acupuncture points or trigger points solely and exclusively intramuscularly are, I think, misinterpreting the simple observations made above.

4 There are some areas of the body where the skin is adjacent to the periosteum, without intervening superficial fascia or muscle layer. Such an area is the medial border of the tibia. If this is pressed when the 'infragenual area' or 'varicose ulcer area' (see Part II of this book) are tender, it will be apparent that the periosteum (as well as the skin) is tender. Hence I think the periosteum is part of the 'tender areas' I describe in this book.

Abbreviations

The following abbreviations might be used on case history cards, particularly by doctors who practice acupuncture a great deal. I would not recommend them for use in other contexts, i.e. books, articles, lectures, etc., where they would be unnecessary and confusing, particularly as in my system of acupuncture usually only one or two needle insertions are required, as opposed to traditional systems which for the most part require greater numbers of needles.

Anterior lateral elbow area	Ale
Anterior medial elbow area	Ame
Anterior superior iliac spine area	Asis
Anterior tubercle of calcaneus	Atc
Cervical articular pillar area	Cap
Dorsalis pedis/dorsal interosseus area	Dpdi
Gastrocnemius tendon area	Gt
Head of metatarsal	Hm
Infraglenoid tubercle	It
Infraorbital foramen area	Iof
Junction of head and shaft of metacarpal	Jhsmc
Junction of head and shaft of metatarsal	Jhsmt
Lambdoid suture area	Ls
Lateral pisiform area	Lp
Lateral process of calcaneal tuberosity	Lpct
Lateral wrist area	Lw
Lumbar spinous processes area	Lsp
Mastoid process area	Mp
Medial infragenual area	Mi
Medial process of calcaneal tuberosity	Mpct

Medial wrist area   Mw
Sacro-iliac joint area   Si
Supraorbital margin/supratrochlear nerve area   Somsn
Trapezius/occiput area   To
Varicose ulcer area   Vu

Index